Talking About Sex in Psychotherapy breaks the silence around one of the most crucial—and most neglected—topics in clinical work. This book makes talking about sex in psychotherapy feel not just possible, but essential. Compelling case studies offer a candid look at the real dynamics and transformative potential of therapeutic work involving sexuality. As someone whose life work was spent training therapists, I recommend this provocative, yet practical, book for training programs and for practicing therapists whose education left the topic of sex unaddressed. Every therapist should read this book because staying silent on this topic can harm our clients.

—**LAURIE MINTZ, PhD,** EMERITUS PROFESSOR, UNIVERSITY OF FLORIDA, GAINESVILLE; AUTHOR OF *A TIRED WOMAN'S GUIDE TO PASSIONATE SEX: RECLAIM YOUR DESIRE AND REIGNITE YOUR RELATIONSHIP* AND *BECOMING CLITERATE: WHY ORGASM EQUALITY MATTERS—AND HOW TO GET IT*

From anecdotal to practical research-supported methodology, this book provides applicable therapeutic intervention through case studies and research. There is a smorgasbord of sexuality topics covered, so that novice and advanced therapists can get something from the chapters.

—**LEXX BROWN-JAMES, PhD, LMFT, CSE, CSES,** DIRECTOR OF THE INSTITUTE FOR SEXUALITY & INTIMACY, LLC, PHILADELPHIA, PA

Drawing on 4 decades of clinical experience with individuals and couples, Kathryn S. K. Hall makes a compelling case for the essential role of open conversations about sex in psychotherapy. She offers thoughtful, practical guidance on how therapists can approach these often sensitive topics with confidence and care. Rich and engaging case examples bring her insights to life, making the book not only informative but also highly readable.

—**CYNTHIA A. GRAHAM, PhD,** DISTINGUISHED PROFESSOR IN GENDER STUDIES AND SENIOR SCIENTIST, THE KINSEY INSTITUTE, INDIANA UNIVERSITY, BLOOMINGTON

Despite sexuality's critical role in the human experience and the prevalence of clients' struggles in this domain, therapists too often avoid conversations with their clients about sex—either because of their own discomfort, limited skills, or a misguided belief in "respect for privacy" regarding sexual issues. Kathryn S. K. Hall offers an essential guide for all therapists who need help *talking about sex in psychotherapy*. This marvelous resource begins with critical foundations for talking with clients about sex—explicating basic principles for prompting the conversation, navigating clients' challenges in the dialogue, and recognizing ethical boundaries. Hall then extends these principles to critical issues such as shame, struggles with sexual desire, sequelae of childhood sexual abuse, and various sexual issues in couple therapy. Enlightened discussion is also devoted to problematic pornography and addressing sexuality with clients in consensually nonmonogamous relationships. *Talking About Sex in Psychotherapy* should be in every clinician's library and will facilitate effectiveness across a broad spectrum of clients with diverse sexual challenges.

—**DOUGLAS K. SNYDER, PhD,** PROFESSOR EMERITUS OF PSYCHOLOGICAL AND BRAIN SCIENCES AT TEXAS A&M UNIVERSITY, COLLEGE STATION; COAUTHOR OF *GETTING PAST THE AFFAIR: A PROGRAM TO HELP YOU COPE, HEAL, AND MOVE ON—TOGETHER OR APART* AND COEDITOR OF *THE CLINICAL HANDBOOK OF COUPLE THERAPY*

Kathryn S. K. Hall offers a clear, concise, and comprehensive guide to understanding and working with sexuality that should be essential reading for all psychotherapists. Moving against the grain of outsourcing this topic to a small group of niche specialists, she provides a state-of-the-art guide to how all therapists can better understand and work with sexuality. Including chapters about ethics, open relationships, kinky sex, couple therapy, and pornography, this is very much a 21st century guide to this work that provides the information that today's therapists need. Well written and filled with illustrative case examples, this book should be in every psychotherapist's library.

—**JAY LEBOW, PhD, ABPP,** CLINICAL PROFESSOR AND SENIOR SCHOLAR, FAMILY INSTITUTE AT NORTHWESTERN AND NORTHWESTERN UNIVERSITY, EVANSTON, IL

TALKING ABOUT SEX IN PSYCHOTHERAPY

TALKING ABOUT SEX IN PSYCHOTHERAPY

A Guide for Every Therapist

KATHRYN S.K. HALL

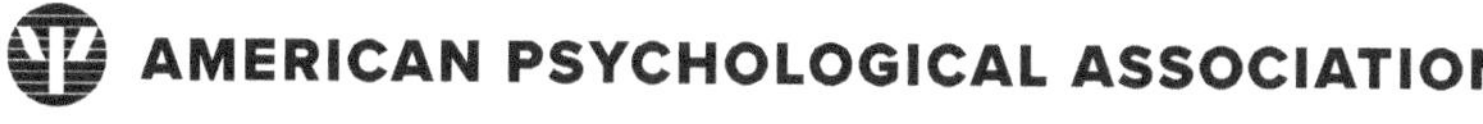

Published by
American Psychological Association
750 First Street, NE
Washington, DC 20002
https://www.apa.org

Order Department
https://www.apa.org/pubs/books
order@apa.org

Typeset in Charter and Interstate by Circle Graphics, Inc., Reisterstown, MD

Printer: Vicks Lithograph & Printing, Yorkville, NY
Cover Designer: Mark Karis

Library of Congress Cataloging-in-Publication Data

Names: Hall, Kathryn S. K. author
Title: Talking about sex in psychotherapy : a guide for every therapist / by Kathryn S. K. Hall.
Description: Washington, DC : American Psychological Association, [2026] | Includes bibliographical references and index.
Identifiers: LCCN 2025015559 (print) | LCCN 2025015560 (ebook) | ISBN 9781433844102 paperback | ISBN 9781433849343 pdf | ISBN 9781433844119 epub
Subjects: LCSH: Sex therapy--Vocational guidance | Psychotherapy patients--Sexual behavior | BISAC: PSYCHOLOGY / Psychotherapy / General | PSYCHOLOGY / Psychotherapy / Couples & Family
Classification: LCC RC557 .H27 2026 (print) | LCC RC557 (ebook)
LC record available at https://lccn.loc.gov/2025015559
LC ebook record available at https://lccn.loc.gov/2025015560

https://doi.org/10.1037/0000483-000

Printed in the United States of America

10 9 8 7 6 5 4 3 2 1

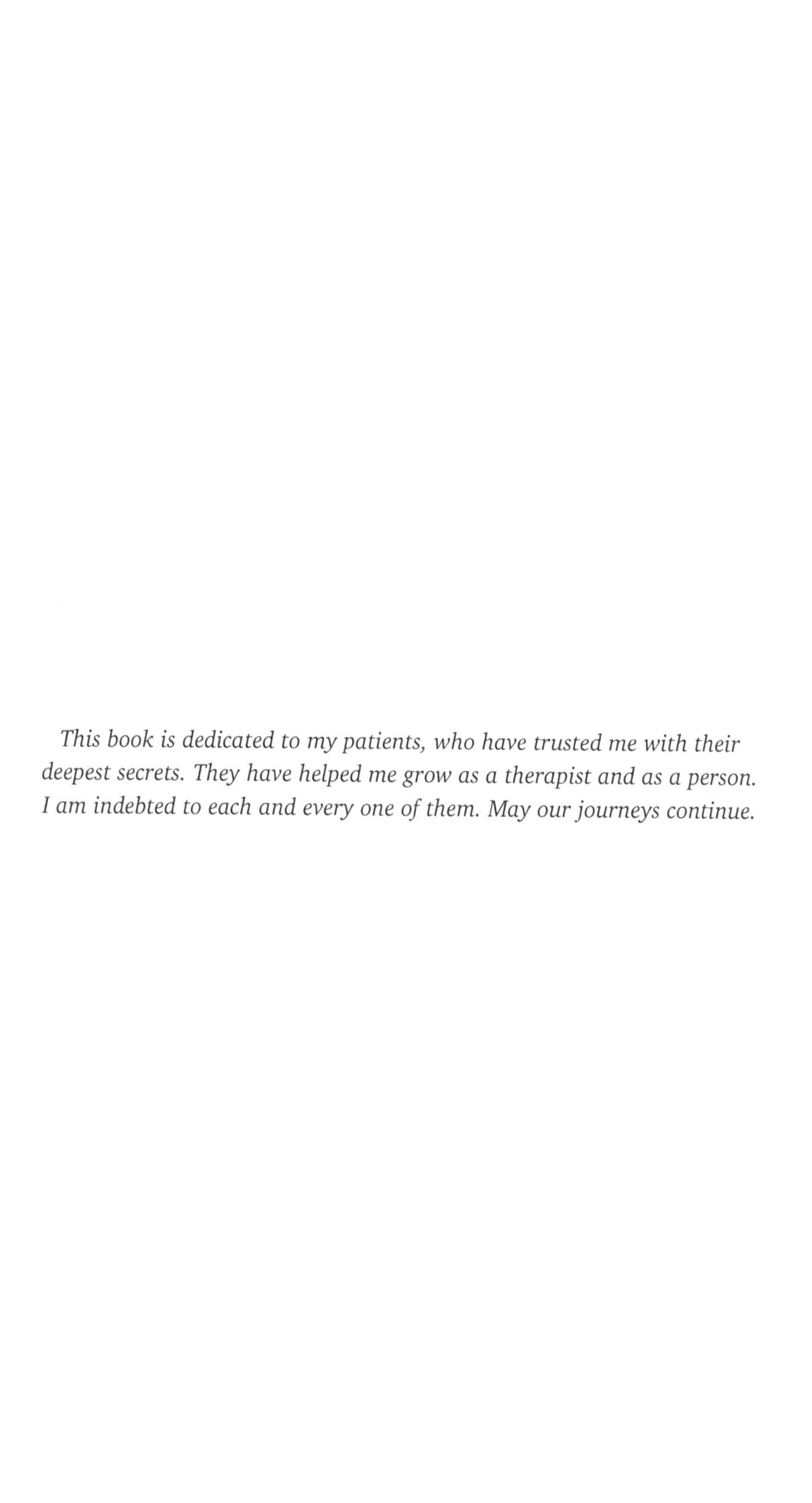

This book is dedicated to my patients, who have trusted me with their deepest secrets. They have helped me grow as a therapist and as a person. I am indebted to each and every one of them. May our journeys continue.

Contents

Acknowledgments

This book represents the culmination of decades of learning. I was well taught by many trusted teachers and clinical supervisors. Three of my mentors deserve special acknowledgment. The late Bill Marshall taught me to be compassionate to those whose sexual behavior was reprehensible. While our sexuality may mirror our internal struggles, he knew that our worst behavior did not define our worth. He was a kind man and an inspirational mentor. The late Sandra Leiblum taught me to be curious without embarrassment and to be unabashedly proud of being a sex therapist. The late Matthew Haar, my clinical supervisor in my fourth decade of clinical work, deepened my love of psychotherapy and encouraged me as I honed my unique style of therapy.

I wanted to write this book for a long time. It took a call from Susan Reynolds, acquisitions editor at APA Books, to get this book out of my head and onto the page. Thank you, Susan, for helping shape this book. My editor, Beth Hatch, got me across the finish line. Beth was seemingly tireless and always enthusiastic and insightful. Thank you, Beth, for your edits, your suggestions, and your guidance. Naomi Burns, copy editor extraordinaire, put the polish on the finished product. Thank you, Naomi, for elevating my writing. A special shout-out to the designer of the brilliant book cover, Mark Karis, so clever and so sassy!

I am forever grateful to have wonderful colleagues in my life, many of whom gave their time and knowledge to help me as I wrote this book.

Special thanks to Laurie Mintz, Irv Binik, Dan Watter, Patricia Hart, Jim Mastrich, Marta Meana, Morag Yule, Patrick Bluett, Michael Vigoritto, and the anonymous reviewers for the American Psychological Association. All of you improved this book. To those whom I am fortunate enough to supervise, please know that you have influenced the way I teach and write about clinical practice. And finally, and sincerely, I give thanks once again to my patients, who inspire me every day to show up and give them my best.

TALKING ABOUT SEX IN PSYCHOTHERAPY

INTRODUCTION

The Importance of Talking About Sex in Psychotherapy

I will confess that I spend a lot of my waking hours thinking about sex. I am, after all, a sex therapist. But this title "sex therapist" is actually misleading. I do not treat sex. I treat people. I treat people who are sexual, which is pretty much everyone. So, I think about and talk about sex in psychotherapy. Talking about sex with my patients helps me and, more importantly, helps them better understand who they are and how they ended up in distress. Sometimes our conversations about sex reveal previously unseen pathways for growth and change. Talking about sex, even when sex is not the presenting problem, can improve the process and outcome of psychotherapy. But talking about sex in psychotherapy is not a skill most clinicians are taught.

I will also confess that talking about sex in psychotherapy was not always easy for me. Explicit conversations about sex made me deeply uncomfortable in the beginning of my practice, but now, not so much, or hardly at all. I have seen how helpful it is, how grateful my patients are for the opportunity to talk honestly about sex, and how therapeutic discussions of sex improve treatment outcomes. In my 40 years of clinical practice, I have learned why and how to talk about sex in psychotherapy. This is what I offer

https://doi.org/10.1037/0000483-001
Talking About Sex in Psychotherapy: A Guide for Every Therapist, by K. S. K. Hall

you in this book: why and how to talk about sex in psychotherapy with all—or almost all—your patients.

Let us begin with a case.

THE IMPORTANCE OF SEX IN PSYCHOTHERAPY

Steve and Amanda came to see me 1 year postdivorce to explore reuniting. After paying a mountain of legal bills and dealing with complex custody arrangements, they surprised even themselves at this turn of events. Steve had gone to therapy and had a breakthrough. The breakthrough had to do with sex. Steve realized that his dissatisfaction with Amanda, his unhappiness that led him to constantly criticize and critique her, started with sexual disappointment.

STEVE: My therapist actually asked me about sex. She asked me if I had been happy with my sex life with Amanda, and she asked me detailed questions about it. That stopped me cold. In all my years in therapy, and when Amanda and I were in couples therapy, no one had ever asked me such questions. And it hit me like a ton of bricks. I remembered constantly wanting Amanda to do oral sex in a particular way, and she never did it. And I remember distinctly having this thought: Is she stupid? Why can't she give me a decent blow job? And so, being the petty bastard that I was, I stopped giving her oral sex, and I began to find fault with her every move, from how she sent text messages to how she managed our finances.

AMANDA: I had no idea he didn't like the way I was doing oral sex. None. I thought I was doing it okay. But I loved when Steve went down on me. And when he stopped, I remember thinking how selfish and lazy he was. And then I couldn't stop seeing him that way, even out of the bedroom.

Amanda and Steve's story demonstrates how permeable the boundary is between sex and other areas of life. And even more than how they thought about each other, they came to see how their sexual problems reflected and reinforced how they thought about themselves. Steve recognized that he often felt he was not getting what he deserved, even though he had difficulty asking. His resentments made him feel petty and mean. Amanda collected and stored grievances, so she often felt aggrieved and therefore unhappy in many of her relationships.

Steve and Amanda's story reflects how talking about sex enriched and enhanced their understanding of themselves and their relationship to each other. (And not to leave you in suspense: No, Steve and Amanda did not reunite, but they are very good coparents and good friends, which they initially were not.) Steve's therapist could not have foreseen the rich therapeutic material that would be uncovered when she asked detailed questions about sex, but she obviously knew it was important to ask. Not all therapists are so inclined.

DISCOMFORT TALKING ABOUT SEX

"As a male therapist, I'm really uncomfortable talking about sex with my female patients." I hear this a lot. In not wanting to cross boundaries or appear predatory or lecherous, male therapists have avoided overt discussions of sex with their (female) patients (except perhaps to note transference). In the wake of the #MeToo movement, which encouraged women to speak out about their experiences of abuse, harassment, and victimization, many of the male therapists who were my colleagues or students worried anew about needing to avoid sexual topics with female patients.[1] They worried about being perceived as inappropriate, about complaints being made against them to their professional boards, or about having negative comments posted on social media. I did not and do not hear the same concern from female therapists. Their reluctance to bring up sex as a topic in therapy is often related to an avoidance of presenting themselves as sexual beings, to avoid bringing attention to their own sexuality. Raising the subject of sex makes many female therapists feel vulnerable; also, they have a vague sense that it is perhaps too "forward."

Many psychotherapists attribute their embarrassment to a lack of training (Emond et al., 2024; Miller & Byers, 2012). Feelings of embarrassment and discomfort are exacerbated in relation to discussing sex with ethnic and sexual minorities, as well as those with intellectual difficulties and older persons (Agochukwu-Mmonu et al., 2021; Dyer & das Nair, 2013). The fear of alienating or offending a patient is sometimes enough to suppress any inquiry. Our own biases may make us think that sex is not a relevant topic for people with intellectual or physical disabilities or for the elderly population. For other

[1]In 2017, #MeToo went viral with people from all walks of life sharing stories of sexual violence, abuse, and harassment. The movement aims to not only help survivors but also disrupt the systems that allow sexual violence to continue (https://metoomvmt.org/get-to-know-us/history-inception/).

patients, we may console ourselves with the thought "Surely the patient will raise the subject if it's relevant." Even those therapists who agree that it is important to discuss sexual issues with patients often fail to do so or to do so routinely (Miller & Byers, 2012). Therapists with issues about their sexuality (questions about their desirability, a history of personal abuse, internalized shame, etc.) certainly will not feel confident saying, "Let's talk about sex."

When patients bring up the topic of sex in therapy, many therapists choose instead to focus on the issues they assume are more important, or more relevant, than sex. I would guess that this maneuver is most often motivated by discomfort, but I might get some opposition to this view. Consider the perspective of Tamika's therapist.

THE RELUCTANT THERAPIST

Tamika sought out therapy postdivorce for help navigating custody arrangements with an irresponsible ex-husband. Therapy helped her be more assertive and to set and hold boundaries with her ex for the sake of their children. When Tamika began to date, she brought the following question to her therapist: "So I really like this new guy I'm seeing, but I never have an orgasm when we're having sex. What do you think this means? I'm worried that I don't really like him like I think I do. Or maybe I'm just not ready for a new relationship?" Her therapist adeptly addressed the latter concern: Was Tamika ready for a new relationship?

The therapist brought this case to my attention during a seminar—to demonstrate that you do not always have to talk about sex. Tamika decided, with the help of her therapist, that she was not quite ready for a new relationship; she had just gotten divorced and had not yet adjusted to being single. According to her therapist, after doing more work examining what went wrong in her marriage, Tamika is now happily dating someone new.

"Yes, it sounds like you have done good work with Tamika. But does she have orgasms with her current partner?" I asked. The therapist confessed he did not know. So, the first time around, the therapist missed an opportunity to explore what Tamika's sexual feelings meant in relation to her emotional connection to herself (readiness to date) and her emotional connection with a partner. This would potentially be an important source of information for a newly single person navigating intimacy and trust in relationships.

In the second instance, by not asking about her sexual experience with her new partner, the therapist also missed an opportunity to let Tamika know that her sexual pleasure was important. And this would again be an important message for any person, but perhaps especially for Tamika and others like her who have difficulty asserting themselves. If Tamika said yes, she was orgasmic, the therapist might or might not explore what this meant in terms of her connection to her emotional state and to this partner. If Tamika said no, she was not orgasmic, the therapist might explore whether this was related to her difficulty asserting herself in relationships and whether and why she was not prioritizing her own pleasure—since it would be very likely that her male partner was having orgasms in all, or at least most, of their sexual interactions (Herbenick et al., 2023). (This could be easily ascertained with a quick question: "Does your partner have an orgasm?")

SEX AS A MIRROR AND MAGNIFIER

By helping our patients explore their sexuality (thoughts, feelings, behaviors) in talk therapy, we are privileged with a new lens that can function as a mirror or a magnifier of underlying psychological dynamics. Steve's marriage did not end because he did not like the way his wife performed oral sex. His sexual dissatisfaction mirrored the way he held on to disappointments and the way those disappointments festered inside him and infected his relationships and his sense of self with bitterness.

Tamika's difficulty having an orgasm during partnered sex postdivorce may mirror her difficulty asserting her own needs and desires in relationships. Holding this mirror up for Tamika may help her see her challenges with assertiveness in a new way and perhaps provide a concrete path for addressing them (for example, helping her advocate for her sexual pleasure with a partner). Tamika's difficulty experiencing orgasm with this particular partner may magnify issues that she may not, at first, notice. Perhaps he is self-centered or just not a skilled lover. Perhaps she is overly worried about his potential disapproval, which distracts her from pleasure. Perhaps when she really cares about a person, she sacrifices her own needs for theirs. We will not know until we ask.

SEX AS A TOPIC IN PSYCHOTHERAPY

In addition to mirroring and magnification, sex is a valid topic in therapy in its own right. It is important to talk about sex in psychotherapy when one considers that almost a third of the general public reports being dissatisfied with their sex life (Heiman et al., 2011; Smith et al., 2011). This percentage is likely higher among those seeking psychotherapy. Many individuals and couples come to therapy because of sexual dissatisfaction, even if they do not identify it as the presenting complaint (Emond et al., 2024). When therapists raise the topic of sex, patients feel they have permission to talk about problems that may be embarrassing or difficult for them to raise, and it signals that the therapist is open to talking about anything and everything in psychotherapy. Additionally, the information we gather about our patients' sexuality provides yet another window into their psychology. Consider the case of David.

David came to see me because he was depressed and procrastinating at work and so not meeting deadlines. He complained that his manager did not spend any time or effort helping him set or meet goals. David had been passed over for a promotion and wanted to "get back on the right track." He described spending a lot of time on his phone and on "random" apps when he should have been doing his work. After several sessions, and with things not quite clicking in therapy, I finally asked David what I should have asked earlier: "What apps are you accessing at work? Dating apps? Porn sites?" Somewhat chagrined, he revealed that he was often on apps looking for a sexual hookup. (David told me that if I had not asked him directly, he likely would never have volunteered this information.) As we talked about his use of apps for sex, it seemed that there was a relationship between his looking for a hookup and disappointment. As we explored the connection, David recounted the following story.

When he was 13, his parents discovered numerous sexually explicit emails between David and an older man. His parents notified the police, and David is not sure what happened after that, but he never heard from this man again. This was a loss for David, as he felt that his email correspondent had been giving him much-needed information about being gay. David's mother responded to the news that her son was gay, and her fear that he was being groomed by a pedophile, by becoming overly protective and smothering. David's father was a different story. David recalls feeling that his father turned cold toward him, and he missed his father's companionship and his previously proffered advice on many aspects of growing up (from cars to fishing and football). He felt he lost his father's love.

Fast-forward to his career, where David again felt the need for guidance from a man, in this case, his manager. When David became anxious at work, he would turn to apps for comfort. He would talk to men on the dating apps until he felt wanted and desired, and this in turn would sexually excite David. Sometimes David would masturbate during the chats, but often he would not. Rarely did he meet up for sex. Usually, once he felt desired, he would simply ghost the man on the other end of the app. Triggered by a feeling of abandonment, David became the one who disappeared and disappointed, rather than being the disappointed one. This insight helped David put down his phone at work and take more responsibility for his work performance, and for his sexual decisions. Parenthetically, it helped him improve his relationship with both parents.

NECESSARY SKILLS

Many therapists do not know what to do when patients raise sexual issues in therapy. What you will discover in reading this book is that for many sexual issues, you already have the necessary skills: listening without judgment, empathic understanding, curiosity, and a genuine desire to work collaboratively with patients toward a resolution that is unique to their situations. When you think of sex as a part—albeit an important part—of the person who is sitting in your office or who appears on your teletherapy screen, you will likely be able to see a connection between your patient's sexuality and their way of being and relating in the world. These insights can help provide direction for working on many of your patient's concerns, including their sexual concerns. These considerations are also highly relevant when you are working with couples. Consider Jane and Hinda.

Jane was genderqueer, identifying as neither male nor female, and was contemplating top surgery. Jane worried that Hinda would either oppose Jane's decision or perhaps end the relationship. After all, she reasoned, Hinda is a lesbian and wants a relationship with a woman.[2] Hinda knew that Jane was considering surgery, but Jane did not talk much about it, so Hinda wanted to respect her privacy and did not talk about it either. In truth, Hinda loved Jane's breasts, and breast stimulation was an important part of her sexual repertoire in past relationships. She hoped that Jane would not have surgery, but she knew that was Jane's decision. Hinda was confident that her love for Jane was not predicated on her breasts.

Neither Jane nor Hinda knew what the other was experiencing, as they did not talk. They came to therapy not because they had ceased to really talk but because they had stopped having sex—irrefutable evidence that something was wrong. As Jane struggled alone with her decision, she became increasingly uncomfortable with sex, and soon this extended to the day or two after sex when Jane would feel depressed and apathetic. Her distress was noticeable to Hinda, as was the change in their sexual activity. Before sex stopped, it became one-sided: Jane pushed Hinda's hands away,

[2]Jane's preferred pronouns continued to be she/her.

she moved her body in ways that made her inaccessible to Hinda, and she focused almost exclusively on bringing Hinda to orgasm while not having an orgasm herself. Hinda was uncomfortable being the only one enjoying sex and found she could not get aroused under these conditions. She worried and waited for Jane to tell her what was wrong. But when that did not happen, Hinda lost her desire for sex as well. And sex between them ceased.

Jane's solution of avoiding sexual arousal mirrored her avoidance of many emotionally difficult subjects. It was not just in their sexual interactions that Jane engaged in avoidance and failed to notice or appreciate Hinda's feelings. Pertaining to other situations, Jane was evasive, defensive, or offered an explanation: "I wasn't avoiding a conversation; I just had work to do." Hinda had difficulty asserting herself and withdrew rather than speaking up. She framed this in her mind as being respectful, as Hinda had suffered through adolescence with incredibly intrusive parents.

The solution, when Jane and Hinda talked openly in couples therapy about their experiences, became obvious to them. Jane asked and learned to trust that Hinda would not touch her breasts during sex. Jane was more vocal about her sexual pleasure but also learned to tell Hinda when she was distressed (even without direct stimulation, sexual excitement made her breasts tingle). They both learned to stay present with each other as Jane regulated her emotional reactions. Hinda learned to advocate for her own pleasure and to speak up when she felt something was wrong. Hinda always knew that she enjoyed sex most when it was mutual, and she became comfortable telling Jane when she preferred to stop or slow down sexually (often, but not always, this was because Jane was uncomfortable).

Together, Jane and Hinda discussed how to manage their sex life while they waited for the top surgery Jane (in conversation with Hinda) finally decided to have. Their strategies included Jane wearing a sports bra and Hinda rubbing or squeezing Jane's legs and feet when Jane was close to orgasm. These strategies took Jane's focus off her breasts and were fun and arousing for Hinda. As they made sexual decisions together, they also began making decisions about other aspects of their life more cooperatively, including the decision about the surgery. They left therapy very satisfied with their relationship and said they would reach out after the surgery if they needed to. I have not heard from them, except for a phone call saying the surgery went well and they are doing "more than fine" and are planning to be married soon.

What I did therapeutically was to be curious, to listen without judgment, to engage in empathic understanding, and then to work collaboratively with Jane and Hinda. Their sex life magnified their poor communication and their use of withdrawal and avoidance as coping mechanisms for stress and conflict. Since sex was the topic that brought them to therapy, I helped them communicate with each other about their sexual experiences and needs, and I encouraged them as they made choices that would lead to more fulfilling sex. Along the way, they were able to use these same skills in other areas of their relationship.

So, here is the question: If sex mirrors and magnifies individual and couples' dynamics, and if working on sexual issues directly can have a positive impact on sex and on other areas of functioning, why are we not taught this as psychotherapists?

MY DISMAL SEX EDUCATION (AND PERHAPS YOURS TOO?)

In my fifth-grade class, we were shown a movie about reproduction. The lights were dimmed, and stick figures appeared on the screen. A dotted line showed the path that sperm took from the male body to the female body, where it met an egg. Nine months later, as a voice-over told us, a baby would be born. The lights came on. My hand went up. None of this made sense to me. Two people stood next to each other and sperm somehow crossed from one to the other? Really? Something important was missing from this story, and I wanted to know what it was.

What was missing, of course, was sex. Without sex, the story I saw in that movie did not make sense. I would suggest that a similar thing happens in psychotherapy (as it did in my work with David). A patient's story, their history, and their presenting problems may not make sense—until you talk about sex, and then the missing pieces appear.

The sex education afforded to psychotherapists is almost as negligible as that of my fifth-grade sex education class. Because there is very little training given to psychotherapists on how and why sexuality is important for understanding and helping patients, you may not feel comfortable talking about sex in psychotherapy, and so you do not. And yet, you have picked up this book because you are at least intrigued by the possibility. And after almost 4 decades of talking about sex with my patients, I want to share those experiences with you. I strongly believe that talking about sex in psychotherapy enriches the process and improves the outcome.

Of course, I was also embarrassed and ashamed of my lack of knowledge in fifth grade. After that experience, I either stayed silent about sex or pretended I knew all there was to know, and laughed at sexual jokes and innuendos in all the right places—when others did. My experience is not unique. There are many ways that we are silenced about sex, and shaming is primary among them; shame about our ignorance, about our own sexual experiences or lack thereof, about having been abused or sexually harassed, and about having perpetrated harassment or pressured someone for sex (telling yourself it was seduction) are some reasons that therapists—who are, after all, people, too—stay silent. Our own therapy and ongoing supervision may be necessary to redress some of these obstacles, but also, you will find guidance in the pages of this book.

But before reading ahead, let me share, briefly, my own journey from silence to sex therapy.

BECOMING A SEX THERAPIST

I started talking about sex by focusing on bad sex. It turns out I am not alone. Many therapists find it easier to talk to patients about the bad sex they have experienced (Cruz et al., 2017). But I am not just talking about bad sex; I am talking about criminal sex. As a practicum student and a research assistant in my undergraduate years, I got my start interviewing incarcerated sex offenders. It was a bit like jumping into the ocean and hoping the sharks have already eaten. In graduate school, I landed an internship doing intake evaluations for a busy sex therapy clinic. Armed with a list of questions I needed to get answered, but with little of my own (clinical or personal) experience, I asked people I had never met and likely would not meet again about the intimate details of their sex lives. Fast-forward over 40 years and thousands of people and patients later, and I could probably talk to almost anyone about their sex life. (Thankfully, I have boundaries, so I do not.) The point is that being comfortable talking about sex with your patients will take time and practice, and the ability to manage your own discomfort in the process. You may start with lists of questions or questionnaires but then eventually learn what and how and when to inquire about sex.

I did not intentionally set out to become a sex therapist. In fact, I think of myself primarily as a psychologist who specializes in helping people with sexual issues. Call me a sex therapist if you need a shorthand version of this title, and I will respond.

BETWEEN THE COVERS: WHAT IS IN THE BOOK?

Therapy is about stories: the stories our patients tell themselves, tell others, and tell us. The stories of the people I have had the fortune to work with grace the pages of this book. I have learned so much from them, and their stories will, I hope, be instructive for you. Names and identifying information are, of course, disguised.[3] Each chapter is anchored by one or two in-depth case discussions to illustrate the principles and techniques being addressed. Sometimes a few briefer cases are included to make a point. Research, which is so important to empirically based practice, is referenced throughout—because working with sexual issues requires that we do not substitute our own preferences and inclinations for what is psychologically healthy for our patients. And research helps us know what that boundary is. Sometimes what we think of as commonsense knowledge is simply not true. Patients have suffered from our ignorance: when they were told that homosexuality was a mental disorder, that having "unusual" sexual interests was deviance, or that their memories of sexual abuse were fantasies and that their clitoral orgasms were manifestations of immature sexual development. Sex research has greatly helped in our understanding of what is "normal," healthy, and even ideal. Happily, sex research is thriving, relevant, and accessible. You will find plenty of it in this book.

The book is divided into two parts. Part I deals with the foundational models underlying the integration of sex and psychotherapy as well as ethical concerns. Part II focuses on integrating sexual issues in the context of psychotherapy. Two appendices outline what you need to know about gendered human sexuality, and the third and fourth appendices provide instructions for sensate focus and a list of sex therapy resources.

THE BOTTOM LINE

Throughout this book I emphasize the importance of good therapy, a strong therapeutic relationship, and an open and nonjudgmental curiosity toward our patients' sexuality. People come to therapy to understand themselves more fully and to resolve whatever issues they are struggling with. Sometimes they will need and want to talk about their sexuality. Therapists have the clinical skills to talk about sex in psychotherapy, to integrate information about their patients' sexuality into a comprehensive and deeper understanding of the person before them, and to helpfully intervene when patients struggle with many sexual issues. It is my hope that this book will provide the inspiration and the blueprint for these endeavors.

It has been a privilege and a pleasure to be privy to the sexual stories of so many people who have trusted me with their secrets. You will notice that

---

[3]All the cases in this book are based on an amalgam of actual cases I have treated. Identifying information has been altered to protect confidentiality.

there are many moments of humor in the therapy examples I give. While sometimes humor is a way of deflecting, it is also a way of joining and sharing. In my years of doing therapy, there have been tears but also laughter, as both are expressions of the deep, healing connection that therapy can bring. It is my hope that you will enjoy reading this book, that you will find some cause to smile when you turn a page, and that you will be touched by the stories of my courageous patients. Whatever wisdom you find in the pages of this book is offered in the hope that it will make the process smoother, by first showing you why it is important to talk about sex and then also offering guidance on how to do that. But most of all, I hope you find this book helpful in your ongoing efforts to deeply and more fully connect with the people who have entrusted you with their care.

PART I FOUNDATIONS

1 THE EVOLUTION OF THE REVOLUTION

Foundational Models of Human Sexuality

[Sex] is admittedly the most important subject in life. . . . It is admittedly the thing that causes the most shipwrecks in the happiness of men and women.

—Watson, 1930, p. 178

John B. Watson, known as the father of behaviorism, believed in the importance of the scientific study of sex so that psychologists might "guide other human beings intelligently" (Watson, 1930, p. 178). But Watson also knew what he was talking about when he was talking about shipwrecks. Watson was himself shipwrecked by sex when his promising academic career was cut short by the revelation of his extramarital affair with his graduate student. Watson never got to study sex but instead found a career in advertising, where he is credited with the invention of the coffee break (Benjamin et al., 2007). Luckily, other sex researchers (not all) have fared better than Watson.

Havelock Ellis, an English physician, is best known for his seven-volume series, *Studies in the Psychology of Sex*, which was published over a 30-year period (1897–1928; Brecher, 1969). This historic work incorporates interviews with his contemporaries, case studies, and cultural insights to address topics as

https://doi.org/10.1037/0000483-002
Talking About Sex in Psychotherapy: A Guide for Every Therapist, by K. S. K. Hall

diverse as modesty, menstrual cycle variations, sexual deviations, venereal disease, multiple orgasms, masturbation, bisexuality, narcissism, and the necessity of sex education. Ellis appeared determined to study sex from a young age, initially perhaps to understand himself more fully but later to help others. Raised in a strict and religious household, Ellis did not masturbate in childhood or adolescence and apparently abstained even into adulthood. At the age of 17, he kept a journal documenting his nocturnal emissions, only to find that they did not increase in frequency and become a progressive disease, as was the commonly held medical belief at the time. This discovery made Ellis question conventional wisdom and further motivated him to study sex.

Nevertheless, Ellis struggled with his own sexuality throughout much of his life. Regardless of having many opportunities, he did not have sexual intercourse until he was in his 30s; he apparently had difficulty having sex with women he loved, and he suffered from premature ejaculation until he was in his 60s. Despite these difficulties, or maybe because of them, *Studies in the Psychology of Sex* is a monumental work wherein Ellis observed the tremendous (normal) sexual diversity among people. After the first of his books was designated obscene in Britain, the remaining six volumes had to be published in the United States with the proviso that they be made available only to members of the medical profession. It is said that his research influenced Freud and anticipated the work of Kinsey and the work of Masters and Johnson, whom I will turn to next (Brecher, 1969).

Alfred Kinsey, a biologist at the University of Indiana, also believed in the necessity of scientifically studying sex in order to better educate his students and prepare them for married life. Kinsey interviewed thousands of Americans about their sexual behaviors, and like Ellis, he documented the extensive scope of sexual behaviors. He had the misfortune, however, to be doing so during the height of the Cold War and McCarthyism. In 1954, after the publication of two books that described the diversity of Americans' sexuality—*Sexual Behavior in the Human Male* (Kinsey et al., 1948) and *Sexual Behavior in the Human Female* (Kinsey et al., 1953)—his funding was cut amid a congressional inquiry into his possible ties to communism. He died unexpectedly 2 years later without ever having secured another funding source.

Ellis and Kinsey are notable for documenting sexual diversity against a backdrop of Victorian morality. They were among the first in a long line of prominent researchers who advocated for accurate, objective, and data-driven information about sex. Subsequently, many others have contributed to the still-growing body of research that more completely informs our understanding of human sexuality. In this chapter, I will review the research and theories that are most foundational for the field of sex therapy and thus most helpful for understanding how and why to integrate sexuality into general psychotherapy. The starting point for our discussion of influential sex research is, of course, the work of William Masters and Virginia Johnson.

SEXUAL LIBERATION: MASTERS AND JOHNSON CHANGE THE WORLD

In sex research, if timing is not everything, it is certainly critically important. And for Masters and Johnson, the timing was right. Although they began studying sexuality in the latter part of the 1950s, their groundbreaking work would not be published until the mid-1960s. The 1960s were a rebellious decade in which young people were intent on upending the status quo: Women were demanding equal rights, the birth control pill made sex without fear of pregnancy possible, and the anti-war protests were converging with the sexual revolution to result in the slogan "Make Love, Not War." The timing was right to liberate sex, not just from the middle-class mores that felt antiquated for the time, but also from the ignorance that left sex a mystery to so many people. For Masters and Johnson, the timing was right, and their collaboration would forever change how the world viewed sexuality and sexual problems.

Timing also dictates what is acceptable research. Masters and Johnson confined their study of sex to the observable and measurable. Most often pictured in white lab coats, they presented themselves as serious medical professionals and scientists. In these professional roles, Masters and Johnson studied the physiology of sex by inviting volunteers into their lab to masturbate or have intercourse while they were observed, filmed, and monitored. On the basis of their scientific observations and measurements, Masters and Johnson laid claim to documenting the human sexual response cycle, a naturally recurring pattern of physiological reactions to sexual stimulation that was experienced by all men and women (Masters & Johnson, 1966). The discovery of nearly identical patterns of male and female sexual responding that followed a predictable linear path from arousal to orgasm was welcome news to the growing feminist movement in the 1960s, as it asserted that women naturally had strong and equal sexuality.

It was good news all around that sex was natural. If sex follows the laws of nature, then there is less that is left to individual choice. Enjoying sex is universal and biological. It is above reproach (Tiefer, 2004). Masters and Johnson, by discovering what was sexually natural, made sex respectable, the study of sex respectable, and the treatment of sexual problems respectable.

The Sexual Response Cycle

The sexual response cycle, as originally described by Masters and Johnson (1966), is depicted in Figure 1.1. The cycle is composed of four phases: arousal, plateau, orgasm, and resolution, which refer to rising sexual excitement, a period of steady levels of sexual arousal, a peak of arousal culminating in orgasm, and then waning arousal as sexual stimulation ceases. The pattern is similar for men and women with a few minor differences. Women are capable of having multiple orgasms (Line A in Figure 1.1) and may also not have any (Line B). Women's arousal may rise and fall quickly (Line C) or may extend for a longer period (Lines A and B). Unlike women, men have a refractory period, a variable length of time needed before it is possible to again become

FIGURE 1.1. Masters and Johnson's Sexual Response Cycle

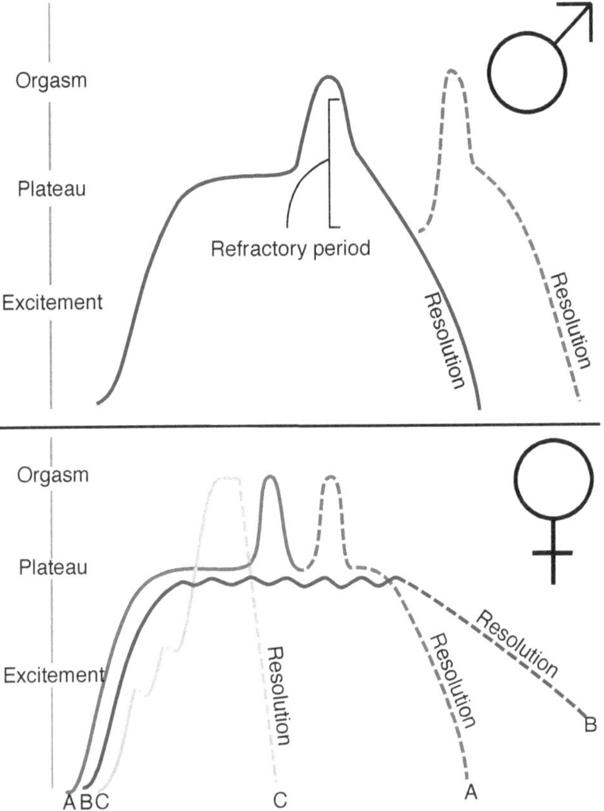

Note. From *Sexual Response Cycle as First Described by Masters and Johnson* [Figure], by Argenti Aertheri, 2023, Wikimedia Commons (https://commons.wikimedia.org/wiki/File:Sexual-response-cycle.svg). CC BY-SA-4.0.

aroused and ejaculate (depicted by the dotted line). I would direct the interested reader, which I hope you are, to Appendices A and B, where you will find more detailed and helpful information on what happens physiologically and anatomically to women and men as they become sexually aroused.

Masters and Johnson's (1966) cycle has been translated from a normative pattern of responding to sexual stimulation to a prescription for providing that stimulation (having heterosexual sex) as well—hence the typical sexual script of foreplay (to get ready), real sex (intercourse), orgasm, and after sex (sleep, cuddle, or the proverbial cigarette). This normative prescription is problematic for many people, and yet many of these same people think this is how they should be doing sex. This normative sexual script is mirrored in our popular culture (the shows we stream, the books we read, the movies and pornography we view). Conformity to this model when it does not quite fit can create problems on its own, as writer Greta Christina (2023) encountered when she tried to count her sexual partners. For example, if you want to sexually stimulate your partner but not get aroused yourself, does that count as sex? What if you do not have an orgasm? Does it count? What if you do not have intercourse? Does it count? What if you mix up the order and have intercourse early and end with caressing and mutual masturbation? Is that wrong? What if you just do not get turned on by the foreplay–intercourse–orgasm model? What if there are two (or more) penises at play? Or no penises at all?

The Creation of Sexual Dysfunctions

Masters and Johnson (1970) followed up on the publication of their first book on sexual responding with a book about sexual problems, rather unfortunately titled *Human Sexual Inadequacy*. In this book they described the malfunctions that could occur at critical stages of the sexual response cycle. Problems with arousal (erectile dysfunction, female arousal disorder) and with orgasm (premature ejaculation, delayed ejaculation, and female orgasmic disorder—which usually implied no orgasms, or no orgasms during partnered sex) became enshrined in the newly created diagnostic category of psychosexual dysfunctions in the *Diagnostic and Statistical Manual of Mental Disorders* (*DSM-III*; American Psychiatric Association, 1980). Also included were two categories of sexual pain disorders: vaginismus (tightening or spasm of the pelvic floor muscles that makes intercourse painful or impossible) and dyspareunia (pain with intercourse either deep in the vagina or at the entrance). These diagnostic categories reflected the gender parity that Masters and Johnson observed in the lab; for example, erectile dysfunction had as its counterpart the rather clumsy and ill-defined category of female arousal disorder, marked physiologically by a lack of vaginal lubrication. The sexual pain disorders were, however, uniquely female.

In addition to documenting problems, Masters and Johnson (1970) also proposed a solution: sex therapy. Masters and Johnson upended years of psychoanalytic tradition in which treatment of sexual problems was focused on resolving underlying conflicts to allow for healthy sexuality to manifest. Masters and Johnson, and subsequent scores of sex therapists, did not and do not consider sexual dysfunctions to be symptoms of deeper conflicts. They consider the sexual dysfunction to be the problem. And according to Masters and Johnson, problematic sex could and should be directly addressed and replaced with pleasurable sex via a series of exercises designed to alleviate the performance anxiety that caused them.

Performance Anxiety

Performance anxiety is defined as excessive worry or concern with sexual performance, marked by the individual monitoring their sexual responses to see if they meet (often unrealistic) standards. This anxious monitoring, or *spectatoring* as it is also called, detracts from the pleasure the individual would otherwise experience and is detrimental to the sexual responding that would otherwise naturally occur. For example, a woman might worry that she is taking too long to reach orgasm. She might start wondering whether her partner is feeling bored or disinterested in stimulating her. She might exhort herself to reach orgasm quickly and focus on her body to see what is going wrong. She might be distracted by worry that she does not measure up to his previous partners. With such heightened performance anxiety, it is highly unlikely that this woman would experience an orgasm. Repeated experiences of failing to achieve the natural and desired result of sexual stimulation (orgasm) would likely make her even more anxious the next time she has partnered sex. Consistently failing to have orgasms during partnered sex would lead to a diagnosis of orgasmic disorder.

The Early Promise of Sex Therapy: Brief, Solution Focused, and Highly Effective!

The sex therapy described by Masters and Johnson (1970) borrowed heavily from behaviorism. In fact, years before the publication of *Human Sexual Inadequacy* (Masters & Johnson, 1970), Joseph Wolpe (1958; Wolpe & Lazarus, 1966) outlined how the principles of learning theory could be used to treat sexual problems, including an intervention that bore a striking resemblance to what Masters and Johnson would later call sensate focus. Masters and Johnson (1970) outlined specific techniques developed for the treatment of specific dysfunctions, but treatment of all the dysfunctions shared some commonalities: psychoeducation about sexual responding and the sexual response cycle, temporarily refraining from sexual activities that cued high anxiety and had high performance pressure (e.g., refraining from intercourse for someone with erectile dysfunction or not engaging in cunnilingus for our fictional female patient with orgasmic dysfunction), and a graded hierarchy of experiences with guidance to focus on pleasure. The most well-known of these interventions is sensate focus, outlined in Appendix C.

Elements of cognitive behavior therapy, just coming into its own in the 1970s, are also evident in Masters and Johnson's (1970) formulation of sex therapy. Sex therapy included directions to replace negative, anxious thoughts with more pleasant and agentic self-talk, instructions and permission to use fantasy and imagery, and techniques to improve both verbal and nonverbal communication during sex (Meana & Hall, 2024). (For those who would like more information on sex therapy for sexual dysfunctions, resources are listed in Appendix D.)

Masters and Johnson (1970) reported impressive results at their treatment clinic, with "success" rates hovering upward of the 90% mark. However, over 50 years later, these outcome statistics have failed to be replicated. This does not mean that sex therapy is an ineffective treatment approach for sexual dysfunctions; it is effective. However, the few rigorously controlled treatment outcome studies show treatment results that do not match the stellar results initially reported by Masters and Johnson. Nonetheless, sex therapy was on the map as a highly specialized and highly effective treatment for sexual dysfunctions. To this day, sex therapy continues to enjoy unprecedented popularity in the public imagination as well as among other professionals (Meana et al., 2020).

A CLOSER LOOK AT THE SEXUAL RESPONSE CYCLE. NOT SO NATURAL AFTER ALL?

Despite the persistence of the universal sexual response model, it does not hold up well under a closer examination of the science behind it. This closer look reveals a biased and imperfect scientific method and calls into question the bold claim of a universal human sexual response cycle. A thorough critique of Masters and Johnson's studies is well documented in Leonore Tiefer's (2004) thought-provoking book *Sex Is Not a Natural Act & Other Essays*. As Tiefer points out, Masters and Johnson assumed the existence of a universal sexual response cycle before they even started their research. They also selected a subject sample that was hardly representative of the general population. Not only were their subjects purposefully weighted toward being of higher-than-average intelligence and socioeconomic status, but also they had a self-professed interest in "effectiveness of sexual performance" (Tiefer, 2004, p. 46), which may account for why they volunteered to have sex while being monitored and watched. It may also account for the finding that performance anxiety was the root cause of sexual problems.

Interestingly, rather than exploring a range of sexual experiences, it was a requirement that both male and female subjects "have a positive history of masturbatory and coital orgasmic experience" (Tiefer, 2004, p. 44). In other words, subjects had to reliably experience orgasm during penile–vaginal intercourse. Having identical performance requirements not only negated the gender difference in masturbatory habits and in orgasmic experiences of the time but also ignored the reality of a gender gap that exists to this day. Men are much more likely than their female partners to have experienced an orgasm during their most recent partnered sex (91% vs. 64%), and this gap widens even further when counting orgasms during sexual intercourse (Herbenick et al., 2023). This seemingly innocuous requirement for participation in Masters and Johnson's studies likely skewed the results and helped perpetuate the belief that most women should be orgasmic from intercourse alone, an erroneous conclusion, as this statistic attests.

By now, many readers will have also recognized the glaring hubris of declaring a universal sexual response cycle when so many people were excluded from the subject pool: people who were not heterosexual; whose gender identity did not fit the binary of male and female; who were older; who were of differing physical abilities, socioeconomic status, and cultural and religious backgrounds; who were self-professed or closet kinksters; and who may not have been aficionados of sexual performance. All these people and many others were not invited to the party and were not counted. It is important to note that homosexuality was still classified as a mental disorder when Masters and Johnson published their findings. It would not be until the revision of the *DSM-III* in 1987 that homosexuality in any manifestation (e.g., a distressing sexual orientation) was no longer considered a mental illness (American Psychiatric Association, 1987). So the universal sexual response cycle is really not so universal after all.

SEXUAL DESIRE: A PROBLEM IN NEED OF A MODEL

It was not long after the introduction of sex therapy that Helen Singer Kaplan (1974) noted a serious problem with Masters and Johnson's model of the human sexual response. There was no beginning; there was no accounting for the motivational state of sexual desire. People were (and still are) coming to sex therapy complaining of a problem that Masters and Johnson's model could not account for: a lack of desire for sex. Kaplan modified Masters and Johnson's model and proposed a triphasic model of sexual responding: desire, arousal, and orgasm.

Problems experiencing sexual desire are currently the most commonly reported sexual complaint among women of all ages. While somewhere between 17% and 33% of women over the age of 65 report low desire, almost half of the women under that age say that their level of desire is problematically low (40%–50%; McCabe et al., 2016). The difference in these age-related percentages is likely due to the fact that low desire is more troubling for younger women than it is for their older counterparts. Despite stereotypes to the contrary, men (ages 18 to 85) also report low sexual desire (19%–28%), with problematically low desire being reported more often by younger men and by gay men (Nobre et al., 2020).

Even though the prevalence of desire problems is relatively high in the general population, simply asking about high, low, or absent levels of desire produces a deceptive picture of the struggles of many people. Sexual desire is complicated and messy. It raises thorny questions about who and what we want (and do not want) sexually. It is so much more than an inborn drive toward orgasm, which was pretty much the best that Masters and Johnson could come up with to explain why people might want to have sex (Tiefer, 2004). Sexual desires may propel one person to kink and another person to the missionary position in the marital bed. Sexual desires are unique. Sometimes desires feel out of control; multiple partners, extended hours watching pornography, and the too-frequent choice of inappropriate partners can result. Sometimes the absence of desire perplexes and hurts people otherwise in love. Our desires can influence how we feel about ourselves and how others view us, and they can affect our very sense of our identity. Desire can and does bring untold pleasure into people's lives. It is why its absence can be so painful.

THE INCENTIVE MOTIVATION MODEL

Masters and Johnson may have neglected to formulate a desire phase of the sexual response cycle because they assumed there was a natural, instinctual drive to have sex. After all, the survival of the human race depends on humans having sex with one another. But humans have a lot more sex than is required for the survival of the species, and much of it has little, if anything, to do with procreation. So why do humans have sex? The short answer might be because it is fun; it feels good. But an additional consideration may be that people have sex because they can.

It turns out that an incentive motivation model may be the most appropriate model to describe human sexual responding. Early animal research revealed that male rodents are not sexually excited or motivated until they are in the presence of a sexually relevant stimulus (a female in heat; Beach, 1956). According to the incentive motivation model, a similar process may apply to human sexual behavior in that one must be in the presence of a sexually relevant stimulus in order to motivate sexual behavior. According to Singer and Toates (1987), some of the main tenets of the incentive motivation model include the following (text in brackets is mine [K. Hall]):

1. Incentives trigger motivated behavior. [If you are in the presence of a sexually attractive person, you will be motivated to seek out some contact with that person.]

2. Incentives inflame motivation by producing affect. [If positive feelings are associated with the incentive, your motivation to be sexual will increase.]

3. Mild deprivation . . . increases the palatability of incentives, broadens the relevant incentive class, and may sometimes produce restlessness. In these senses we might speak of "drive-like" effects of deprivation. [If you cannot be with the one you love, love the one you are with.]

4. The hedonic quality of particular incentives is decreased by constant use or consummation and enhanced by abstinence from that particular incentive. [In other words, distance makes the heart grow fonder.] (pp. 484–485)

If drive is defined as "the 'push' of motivation, a goading internal state that exists even in the absence of an external incentive" (Singer & Toates, 1987, p. 483), then there is no evidence of a sex drive in humans.

Clinicians will have noted the folly of believing that sex is a drive (like hunger) when they have observed in couples that the strategy of the higher-desiring partner withholding sex in the hopes of encouraging a low- or non-desiring partner to initiate is most often a failing proposition. It may work with food; hunger will eventually propel someone to eat, even food that is not that delicious. But it does not work for sex. My patient Rick decided that he would not initiate sex with his wife until she initiated sex with him. He was tired of being rejected, and he felt certain that once she knew how it felt to go without sex, once her sex drive kicked in and she felt deprived, she would be coming on to him with apologies in hand. Rick dedicated a whole year to his experiment: "When will she notice? When will she want me?" Sadly, for Rick and for his wife, all that happened was that Rick spent the year seething with barely hidden resentment. If his wife noted the lack of sex, she may have attributed it to many things (his bad mood, fatigue, distractions, age). Or, she may have felt relieved. What Rick failed to understand was that a seething, resentful husband is not an ideal incentive for sex. And there needs to be an incentive to motivate sexual behavior.

BASSON'S CIRCULAR MODEL

Rosemary Basson (2001), a gynecologist in British Columbia, Canada, noticed something important as she listened to the sexual experiences of her patients. What motivated her patients to be sexual was not, primarily, a desire for sex. Her model of sexual responding, known as the circular model for obvious reasons, is depicted in Figure 1.2. In this model, sexual behavior can begin from a position of sexual neutrality. In the earliest iterations of this model, the wish to be more emotionally intimate with a partner sets the motivation to seek or be receptive to sexual experiences. This allows for the possibility of those experiences to be sexually arousing, which leads to a desire for more sexual stimulation and arousal.

FIGURE 1.2. Basson's Circular Model of Sexual Response

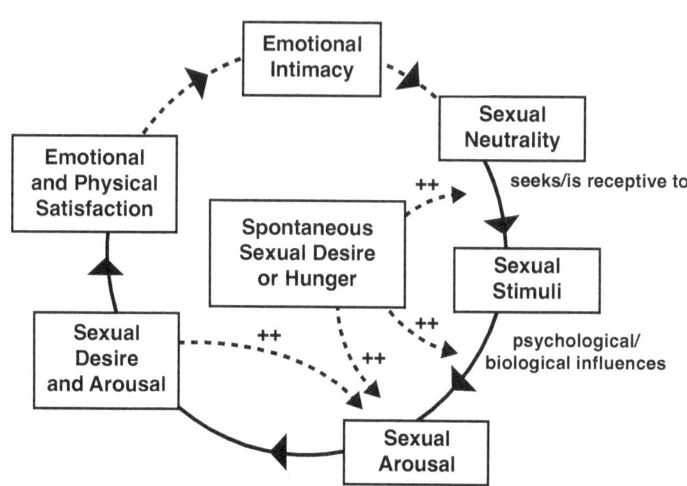

Note. From "Human Sex-Response Cycles," by R. Basson, 2001, *Journal of Sex & Marital Therapy*, *27*(1), p. 38 (https://doi.org/10.1080/00926230152035831). Copyright 2001 by Taylor & Francis. Reprinted with permission.

Sexual desire kicks in when sexual arousal begins and then desire and arousal engage in a mutually enhancing feedback loop: Arousal leads to the desire for more sexual stimulation, which increases arousal, and so on. The idea that desire is not just a preliminary phase of a linear model of sex was truly revolutionary (Basson [2001] noted that there was nothing inherently cyclical about Masters and Johnson's sexual response cycle). You do not have to feel desire in order to initiate or agree to sex! You just have to be open to the possibility of sex and sexual pleasure. Desire should accompany arousal throughout sexual activity, providing the ongoing motivation to keep on going. Sexual satisfaction results from not just orgasm or heightened arousal but also the emotional satisfaction of being intimate. The pleasure that results enhances the motivation to seek or be receptive to sexual activity in the future.

This circular model, now widely known as Basson's (2001) circular model, reflects the lived experience of many people, especially women. Thanks also to some focused research, demonstrating that for many women the states of desire and arousal are indistinguishable (Graham et al., 2004, 2006), the fifth edition of the *Diagnostic and Statistical Manual of Mental Disorders* (*DSM-5*; American Psychiatric Association, 2013) has departed from the tradition of having the same categories of sexual dysfunctions for men and women. As of 2013, the category of hypoactive sexual desire disorder has stayed in place for men but for women was replaced with a new diagnostic category of female sexual interest/arousal disorder, which merged low desire with female sexual arousal dysfunction.

Basson's (2001) model also provides for the possibility that sexual activity can be motivated by spontaneous sexual desire. Men, in general, do distinguish desire from arousal, perhaps because they are accustomed to having erections when they are aroused, and so they have an observable line of demarcation, as it were. Men resonate with the idea that they feel spontaneous and physical manifestations of the wish for sex. Basson notes that this state of sexual hunger (as she refers to it) occurs most often in younger people and motivates them to seek out sexual opportunities. This inner cycle that starts with desire is similar to the sexual response cycles of Masters and Johnson (1966) and Kaplan (1974). Key, however, to Basson's (2001) model is that sexual activity is constantly being processed by the mind (awareness) and experienced by the body in a reciprocal feedback loop such that an awareness of pleasure becomes physically stimulating, which increases the awareness of pleasure . . . and so on until time, energy, or orgasm provides an end point.

Sexual problems can arise when this cycle is interfered with. For example, psychological or biological factors can inhibit the processing of sexual stimuli so that arousal does not occur and the cycle does not continue. Psychological factors may include anxiety, depression, relationship distress, or the blunting of pleasure from past traumatic experiences. Biological factors can include depression, medication side effects, fatigue, or hormonal imbalances. If sexual and emotional satisfaction does not result from sexual activity, whether due to psychological or biological inhibition, or because the resulting sex was painful or disappointing, the motivation to seek or be receptive to sex in the future will be weakened. Relationship distress or difficulties will likewise interfere with the cycle, inhibiting the initiation of sex or diminishing the intimacy and emotional satisfaction that would otherwise result.

A CLINICAL EXAMPLE OF CIRCULAR RESPONDING

Maeve and Fred are 28 and 27 years old, respectively. They have one child, an active 3-year-old boy named Sam. It was difficult for Maeve and Fred to get their sex life back on track after Sam was born, and they found themselves arguing a lot. The stress of juggling work and parenting was challenging, especially for Maeve. Maeve wanted more help with household tasks and childcare, while Fred wanted to go on dates and have a more active sex life. They came to therapy full of resentment. Maeve resented Fred for not helping out more, and Fred resented Maeve for not prioritizing their relationship. As they talked in therapy, they realized that their goals were similar: to improve their relationship. It is just that they imagined different paths to the same end. As Fred came to understand Maeve's point of view, he agreed to be more proactive in doing household tasks. He recognized that although he can do tasks without really feeling like it, he cannot expect Maeve to have sex with him when she does not want to.

One day, as Fred was playing with Sam and teaching him a fun game of clean up the living room, Maeve noticed tender feelings for Fred. She drew him aside and kissed him. She was motivated to do this because she felt close to him. Fred was encouraged, and after Sam went to bed, he offered to give Maeve a back rub. She agreed, as she wanted the close feelings she had to continue. She knew the back rub could lead to sex, and she was open to it. As Fred was rubbing her back, Maeve noticed that she was beginning to get aroused. She liked the feeling and was open to more caressing and kissing. As Maeve became aroused, she took an active role in stimulating Fred, which made her feel sexy. The sex they had was enjoyable, and they felt emotionally close to one another and sexually satisfied. There was a high likelihood that Fred and Maeve would have sex again in the future.

Their progress was disrupted when Maeve felt too exhausted to have a planned date night with Fred. Fred was disappointed and felt like this was the same old story. He made his disappointment obvious. Maeve felt guilty and decided to just go ahead and have sex to make Fred happy. So, they started having sex. But Maeve was not into it. She was resentful that she had to have sex with Fred despite her tiredness, and she was angry at him for not noticing her fatigue. "All he wants is sex," she thought. During sex Maeve started thinking about her mother, who essentially waited on Maeve's father hand and foot. Maeve swore she would never be like her mother, and the thought came to her that here she was, having sex so her husband would not be upset. Weak. Just like her mother. Maeve's body was not responding to Fred's touches. Her mind was elsewhere. She wanted Fred to hurry up and finish. The sex was disappointing and somewhat painful for the unaroused Maeve. Fred was perplexed and confused. Maeve said yes to sex, and yet she did not even try to enjoy it. He felt vaguely foolish and embarrassed. The likelihood of sex in the future was diminished.

The desire–arousal feedback loop did not kick in once Maeve and Fred started to have sex. Maeve was not really in a place of neutrality to start with; she was exhausted and did not want to have sex. Maybe Maeve deserves kudos for trying because she might have enjoyed the sex once it started. But when Maeve knew her body was not responding and that she really was not going to enjoy the experience, she should have stopped right then. This would ultimately have been better for both Maeve and Fred. Consensual but unwanted (and therefore unpleasant) sex, if it occurs too often, can lead to sex becoming an aversive experience. Maeve might well have said, "I need to sleep; this is not working for me tonight." And yes, Fred would have been disappointed. But in the context of a good sex life, disappointments can be expected, and tolerated, from time to time.

NOT ALL MOTIVATIONS FOR SEX ARE EQUAL

While the wish for emotional intimacy was initially highlighted by Basson (2001) as the starting point for sex, there is currently a recognition of other nonsexual motivators that move individuals from sexual neutrality to sexual behavior. In a large-scale study examining why humans have sex, Meston and Buss (2007) documented 237 distinct motivations ranging from the physical (pleasure, stress reduction, experiencing-seeking) to the emotional (love, commitment), the utilitarian (social status, revenge, access to resources), and the psychological (self-esteem boost, insecurity, duty/pressure). Follow-up studies have examined how sexual motivation is influenced by age (Meston et al., 2009), gender, and sexual function (Meston & Stanton, 2017; Stephenson et al., 2011).

What motivates people to be sexual (partnered or solo) is intricately related to the role that sex has played in their life, their history, their current psychological dynamics, their relationship status, and their very sense of themselves. But as we saw with Maeve and Fred, not all motivations lead to good sexual experiences, because not all motivations truly signal an openness to giving and receiving sexual pleasure.

THE PUSH AND PULL OF SEX: THE DUAL CONTROL MODEL

The idea that there are incentives that pull on sexual desire as well as factors that inhibit desire has been part of the mainstay of many theories of sexuality. Certainly, psychoanalytic theory emphasizes the underlying conflicts that push and pull people between wanting to satisfy their desires and believing (accurately or not) that they cannot or should not. Without referencing underlying drive states or other psychoanalytic concepts, the idea that there are essentially two systems—excitatory and inhibitory—in terms of sexual responding was convincingly described by John Bancroft and Erick Janssen (2000) from the Kinsey Institute, and was named the dual control model of sexual response.

In her popular book *Come as You Are*, Emily Nagoski (2021) translated the science for the lay public when she described competing impulses as brakes and accelerators. Brakes and accelerators are unique to the individual and to their relationships. Brakes are things that are colloquially referred to as *turnoffs*, such as bad breath, sarcastic remarks, and children awake in the next room. Accelerators are *turn-ons* and may be things like compliments, a muscular physique, flirtation, or an erotic caress. People may have an abundance of brakes and very few accelerators and so find it difficult to be in the mood for sex. The converse, very few brakes and many accelerators, can lead to frequent and indiscriminate sexual behaviors.

In our offices, or on our teletherapy screens, our patients share their struggles with the push and pull of competing interests when it comes to sex. For Maeve it was about not wanting to disappoint Fred while also wanting to hold onto a fundamental belief she held about herself: "I am a strong woman. I am not like my mother." For others, the tension of competing desires may have to do with infidelity, confusion about sexual orientation, or enjoyment of (kinky) sex that is at odds with their moral code or religious beliefs.

TODAY'S UMBRELLA MODEL: THE BIOPSYCHOSOCIAL MODEL

We find ourselves now understanding that sex is more than the physical responses described by Masters and Johnson (1966). It is driven not by an instinctual need for sex or orgasm but by sexual and nonsexual incentives. We have moved beyond acknowledging performance anxiety to note that how one thinks about, feels, and responds to their sexual responding (which can be both positive/enhancing and negative/inhibiting) is important.

All the models previously discussed—Masters and Johnson's (1966) sexual response cycle, the circular model (Basson, 2001), the incentive motivation model, and the dual control model (Bancroft & Janssen, 2000)—fit under the umbrella of a biopsychosocial understanding of human sexuality. This means that regardless of the flavor, the sex referred to in all our models of sexual responding relies on a combination of factors working together, including biological (e.g., hormonal, physiological, anatomical), psychological (e.g., mental health issues such as anxiety or depression, body image concerns, attachment style, trauma history), social (e.g., family of origin and cultural and religious influences), and interpersonal (e.g., relationship distress). A problem in just one area (e.g., the relationship distress of Maeve and Fred) is often enough to disrupt sexual functioning, although due to the overlapping nature of the factors in the biopsychosocial model, problems usually occur in more than one domain. Problems also arise when there are conflicts, say, between biological factors (strong sexual interest) and psychological issues (e.g., anxiety), such that there is a push (I want to) and a restraint (I am afraid). Comprehensive treatment of sexual difficulties usually requires addressing multiple domains.

And this puts us squarely back into terrain that is familiar to most psychotherapists—the landscape of our patients' thoughts, feelings, anxiety, and the competing demands of their current life situation as well as family of origin issues and histories of trauma.

WAIT, WHAT IS SEX ANYWAY?

Before we move on to talk about integrating discussions of sexuality into ongoing psychotherapy, we need to understand, or at least agree upon, what sex is. All the models we have discussed so far have described how sex works (and does not). But if we harken back to the beginning of the chapter and the dilemma experienced by the writer Greta Christina (2023) as she tried to determine what counted as sex, we realize that we are sometimes faced with a definitional issue.

Sex is often defined by the social conventions of the time. Social norms, rather than empirical data, have long determined what sexual behaviors are considered normal or healthy. Historically, that has meant that procreative sex was considered to be sex, and the rest was deviance, or in scientific parlance, a *paraphilia*.

In Latin, *para* means next to or adjacent to, and *philia* means love. So, literally, paraphilias are those behaviors that are additional, such as the cherry on a sundae or the extra shot of espresso in your morning coffee. They are not strictly necessary for love (sex) but are desirable. In practice, however, paraphilia has come to take on negative connotations, with the meaning of not just next to but also atypical, abnormal, unhealthy, and deviant. (See Chapter 7 for a more detailed discussion of kinky sexual interests.)

It turns out, however, that when we do look at the data, there is nothing atypical or unhealthy about these adjacent sexual activities. Studies have failed to find a link between any particular sexual interest (not including criminal behavior) and psychopathology (Joyal, 2021). And yet, therapists may mistake their own discomfort about certain expressions of sexuality for their clinical judgment that it is unhealthy. Consider the story of April and Joe.

A LOVE STORY SET IN A SEX CLUB

Joe met April at a sex club. She was there with her abusive husband, who had watched (and masturbated) while she and Joe had sex. But April and Joe felt a connection (he had noticed her bruises and was tender with her), and they continued their relationship outside of the club and away from her husband's sexualized gaze. April eventually got divorced with the hope of being in a relationship with Joe, but he was having difficulty leaving his marriage. Joe came to therapy to understand why he remained in an unhappy marriage when he really wanted to be with April. Joe and April continued to go to sex clubs where they had sex with each other and with other partners. A few months into his therapy with me, April's therapist called. Could Joe really be a good choice for April given that he took her to sex clubs? The therapist believed that April had left one abusive relationship for another. April's therapist made a mistake that therapists often make. She judged Joe based on his sexual preferences without adequate knowledge about sexuality, or about Joe. She pathologized his sexual behavior, and then she pathologized him. April's first husband was abusive, and he enjoyed going to sex clubs. Joe was a responsible and loving man (contributing to his difficulty in leaving his unhappy marriage), and he enjoyed going to sex clubs. April had been in an abusive marriage, and she enjoyed going to sex clubs. Going to sex clubs was a common denominator, but it was not the problem for April and Joe.

Had Joe come to therapy decades earlier, the therapist might have felt the goal was to help Joe give up his affair and be happy in his marriage. And Joe might well have agreed, swayed by the social stigma of divorce. Furthermore, the therapist might have felt that Joe's interest in having sex in sex clubs was evidence of not just deviant sexuality but also psychopathology: "You can't make a commitment, so you pursue anonymous sex. You hate women, so you engage in anonymous sex. You hate men, so you have sex with their wives in front of them. You feel inadequate." And Joe might have been convinced. But Joe came to see me only a few short years ago, and he was pretty confident that there was nothing pathological about the pleasure he experienced at sex clubs. In fact, Joe chose to see a sex therapist because he felt hopeful that his sexuality would be understood and not pathologized. He wanted the focus in therapy to be on understanding his inability to leave his marriage.

Joe came to therapy to resolve a conflict. Part of him wanted to be with April, but another part of him felt duty bound to stay with his wife. Unpacking and understanding his dilemma started by talking about sex. As you will see in the many cases in this book, talking directly about sex can provide a useful tool to propel therapy. Sex, as it was in Joe's case, can be a mirror, a reflection in sharp focus, of who Joe is and what his struggles are about. This is what I asked: "Joe, tell me how you feel when you are at the sex club with April."

Joe described feeling proud, proud to be there with a beautiful woman. He felt proud to be an attractive and sexual man, and he enjoyed knowing people were watching him. He felt responsible for making sure that April was safe and happy. It added to his pleasure that he was looking out for her. He felt the freedom to have sex (or not) with whoever he desired and whoever desired him. He felt proud, loving, responsible, and liberated at the same time. In this context he felt sexual and happy. In his marriage, Joe described feeling a heavy sense of duty and responsibility. He had no sexual desire for his wife, and it seemed that she had none for him. It had been years since they last had sex.

What I learned from Joe's sexual experiences helped me to focus on the role that duty, shame, pride, and sex played in Joe's life. He recounted being raised by a single mother who was an alcoholic. They were poor, and Joe felt a great deal of shame about their circumstances. From the time he was in grade school, Joe was responsible for taking care of his mother. Sometimes that meant getting her home from a bar where she had either become unruly or passed out. He knew before he was old enough to truly understand that his mother often left the bar with men she met there. Joe felt trapped growing up, trapped by shame and responsibility.

Joe was always seeking a balance between responsibility and freedom. He erred on the side of being responsible (and sexually and morally upstanding) when he married his wife. Joe's wife, in Joe's estimation, was a kind and good person who nonetheless always saw the bleak side of life. His wife, he came to realize, suffered from anxiety and depression but, to his great disappointment, did not want to change. She wanted Joe to take care of her. During his marriage Joe may have found a workable balance between responsibility and freedom by going to sex clubs on occasion and tending to his wife and family the rest of the time. But then, years later, he met April. A new balance now seemed possible, as Joe had tender and caring feelings for April as well as a sense of freedom and possibility. Leaving his marriage may have felt possible, as Joe thought perhaps he had completed his duty to his wife, having seen their youngest child graduate from college. Viewing his struggles as a quest for balance between his sense of duty (which might have been overdeveloped from childhood) and the freedom he craved helped Joe ultimately decide to leave his marriage.

Understanding Joe's sexuality in the context of his life was important. Going to sex clubs meant something different for Joe than it likely does for others. His unique sexual experiences reflected important dynamics in his life, with relevance to his struggles.

In a tragic turn of events, April was killed by a drunk driver shortly after Joe left his wife. April and Joe were people who struggled to reconcile their caring natures with their spirit of adventure. In sex clubs they found the freedom and adventure they craved and enjoyed. And even if only briefly, they found each other.

SUMMARY

Our current understanding of the complexity of sex has grown beyond Masters and Johnson's (1966) model of a universal sexual response cycle. There is not just one model of sexual responding but several models that complement each other. The biopsychosocial model provides an overall perspective on sexuality, highlighting the fact that biological, psychological, sociocultural, and interpersonal factors all contribute to sexual functioning and pleasure. Our understanding of sexual desire has changed from the idea of an internal drive state to an incentive motivation model, with clinical applications described and depicted by Basson's (2001) circular model of sexual responding. Desire, as we now know, is not just a prerequisite motivational state but also a force that dynamically interacts with sexual arousal throughout sexual activity. The dual control model (Bancroft & Janssen, 2000) highlights the push and pull of competing interests (excitatory and inhibitory factors) on sexual arousal and desire.

An appreciation of these foundational models will shape the clinical conversations we have in therapy. The cases described in this chapter illustrate how sex can be a mirror and a magnifier of important personal and interpersonal dynamics. The story of Joe and April also reminds us that atypical sexual experiences can mirror and magnify important issues in our patients' lives and that we can discuss atypical interests in therapy without pathologizing them.

2 HOW TO TALK ABOUT SEX IN PSYCHOTHERAPY

It may not feel very intuitive to ask about sexuality in preliminary meetings with many of our patients. For example, when Tamika (whom we met in the Introduction) came to therapy for help setting boundaries with her ex-husband, it might have felt to her like a boundary violation for her therapist to have asked about her sex life. This issue would have been further complicated by the fact that her therapist was a white male and Tamika was African American. Black women have historically had their sexuality questioned, fetishized, and misinterpreted. The Jezebel stereotype of a lascivious, innately promiscuous, and even predatory seductress continues to haunt Black women to this day (Leath et al., 2021; West, 1995). The reluctance of Tamika's therapist to ask questions about her sexuality is understandable. Or take my treatment of David, a gay man in his late 20s (also outlined in the Introduction). He came to therapy for help with depression and procrastination. However, when David reported wasting time on the internet, my failure to ask in a timely fashion about sexual content in his internet use was overly cautious, perhaps influenced by my misguided effort not to feed into the stereotype of the promiscuous gay male.

https://doi.org/10.1037/0000483-003
Talking About Sex in Psychotherapy: A Guide for Every Therapist, by K. S. K. Hall

In psychotherapy, therapists often rely on their clinical intuition to help them know when and how to ask questions about various topics. But how do we rely on our clinical intuition when asking questions about sex given that we are not taught or encouraged to do so and when, as the above examples illustrate, other biases may be at play? Most often our training on sex and psychotherapy, if any, admonishes us not to consider our patients as sexual beings lest we cross a boundary and have sex with them. But as many of the cases in this book illustrate, it is possible, perhaps even ideal, to see our patients as sexual beings without crossing boundaries. Clinical intuition takes time and practice, so I will offer a few guidelines in the interim.

ASKING ABOUT SEX DURING AN INITIAL ASSESSMENT

If you take a thorough history at the beginning of your work with patients, here are some guidelines on incorporating questions about sex. And if you do indeed conduct a thorough history, questions about sex should become a routine part of your inquiry. Otherwise, you are not truly doing a thorough history. Note that during an initial assessment, the reason you are asking about sex is the same reason you are asking about any number of things in the patient's life and past: You are getting to know the patient, and you are casting a wide net to see what and where the problems (and strengths) might be in order to formulate a treatment plan.

Inquiring about sex at these early stages of therapy and assessment has these important additional benefits: Understanding a patient's sexuality helps you to understand how they relate intimately (or not) to others, how they manage boundaries, and how they relate to their own body. Recall that sex can mirror and magnify many psychological issues. Bringing up the topic of sex early on in therapy also signals to the patient that you are open to discussing sex (so it is easier to talk about it later if relevant), and since you can talk about sex, you are signaling that you can talk about almost any topic in therapy. Here are some ways to ask about sex in the context of other common topics.

Family of Origin Issues

When discussing family of origin, you can uncover a lot about communication and boundaries by asking about sex: "How was the communication in your family—for example, who told you about sex, or how was sexuality discussed in your family?" "What were the sleeping arrangements in your home?" "What messages did you get about intimacy and sexuality from the fact that __________ [your parents didn't sleep together/doors had to be left open/you could always (or could never) sleep in your parents' bed/your brother's significant other could sleep over in his room but your significant other had to go home, etc.]?" Information about marriages, divorces, infidelity, and infertility issues can provide insights into sexual messages and values that are transmitted intergenerationally.

Developmental History

Important milestones are opportunities to ask about sex. This helps you understand the impact of these milestones on the patient's ability to be intimate, on their relationship to their body, and whether and how they might use sex as a coping mechanism (in the positive, neutral, or negative sense). Asking about their first sexual experience can help you understand how they related to their peer group. Asking about how they became aware of their own sexuality helps you better understand their relationship to themselves. I might ask, "How did you first learn about sex?" or "When did you first become aware of your sexuality?" Other questions can include "When did you start to explore your own body?"; "When did you begin to masturbate?"; and "How did you learn about masturbation?" These questions can also reveal inappropriate or abusive experiences, even if the patient does not label them as such.

Inquiry about sex when exploring how your patient adjusted (or did not) to significant changes (coming out, beginning to date, pregnancy, miscarriage, marriage, cohabitation) can further your understanding of how the patient regulates their emotional state. For example, when the frequency of sex or sexual desire diminishes with what Dan Watter (2023) calls *relationship-deepening events* (cohabitation, marriage, engagement), we can understand this as a reaction to commitment and/or intimacy. For example, many couples come to therapy perplexed as to why their perfectly happy sex life disappeared when they moved in together. Some people adjust to divorce or the ending of a relationship or infidelity by shutting down emotionally (no sex) or needing to have validation that they are still desirable (having an increase in the frequency of sex or in the number of sex partners).

Traumatic Experiences

Asking "Have you had sexual experiences that were confusing, traumatic, or that you regretted?" can lead to the disclosure of negative or abusive sexual experiences. If you know from asking or from the patient's self-report that there were sexual or other forms of abuse in childhood, ask directly, "How has that experience affected your sexuality?" You will want to inquire about several time points: in the immediate aftermath, in adolescence, and later in adulthood. I typically start with open-ended questions and then provide helpful prompts if the patient does not answer. When prompting, I give an array of options so the patient knows that any answer they give is acceptable: "Some people find there is no impact, whereas others find they are disconnected from sex later in life, they have a lot of sex (or none at all), they enjoy a lot of sex, or they dislike the sex they do have. Do any of these reactions resonate with you?" If the abuse was not sexual, the questions are still valid: "Experiences like the ones you describe often affect the ability to trust, to enjoy your own body, or to be intimate with others." Pause and listen to the answer; if there is no overt discussion about sexuality, ask the follow-up: "How did those experiences affect your sexuality?"

The same logic and format of questioning may follow from other experiences that would intuitively relate to sex: infertility, fertility treatments, infidelity, divorce, and difficult breakups. It is a relevant follow-up question to ask, "How has the difficulty of [conceiving/going through a contentious divorce/this breakup] affected your sexuality?" As with other inquiries, asking about masturbation may need to be explicit, as many patients will assume that questions about sex refer only to sexual interactions with others: "So sex with your partner was difficult. What about sex with yourself—masturbation?" Differentiating partnered versus solo sexual experiences can clarify relational issues (e.g., attachment anxiety).

Current Relationships

Most assessments will involve exploring the patient's past and current relationships. This, of course, provides an excellent opportunity to ask about sex, as it will help clarify relationship dynamics. Understanding sexuality as a mirror and a magnifier is very helpful at this point in the inquiry. If the patient says they are currently in a relationship and you ask about the relationship, you can also explicitly ask, "How would you describe your sexual relationship with __________?"

Let us go back to Tamika. Imagine that the subject of sex, namely, her lack of orgasms with her current partner, arose during an initial evaluation. If instead of deciding that the more important or immediate topic to discuss was her readiness to date, what if her therapist had stayed on the subject of sex?

THERAPIST: You don't have orgasms with Bob? Is that unusual for you when you have sex with a partner?

TAMIKA: Oh yes, usually I am really excited during sex, and I cum pretty easily. Not always or even usually with sex, but with oral, or if he uses his hand.

THERAPIST: Why do you think you don't cum with Bob?

TAMIKA: Well, one pretty obvious reason is that he doesn't seem to notice, or maybe he doesn't care that I haven't cum, but I don't know why I don't tell him. Usually I do. Usually I'm pretty specific with my partners about what I want.

THERAPIST: So this is why you are confused—you're not sure why you are not telling Bob that you haven't had an orgasm, or asking for some stimulation from him that would bring you to orgasm.

TAMIKA: Right! Why is that? There's nothing special about Bob. I'm not really sure I like him that much.

THERAPIST: Hmm. So you are having sex that is not so great for you with a guy you're not sure you really like all that much.

TAMIKA: Well, when you put it that way . . . maybe I am rushing things.

THERAPIST: It would seem that your body is telling you that you are not really invested in this relationship with Bob.

From here, the discussion might center on why Tamika was pushing herself. Questions might focus on what psychological needs are being met by being in a relationship with Bob, what social or cultural forces are at play (Is it culturally important for her to have a partner?), and what the interpersonal dynamics are between her and Bob that have led her to have sex that is not very pleasurable for her. We might come to understand Tamika as being lonely, feeling rejected by her ex-husband, or wanting to prove that she is desirable (a psychological factor). Or we might find that being a single Black woman with children exposes her to social criticism, that in her family it is important to be partnered with a man (a cultural and social factor), or that with Bob, in particular, Tamika is deferring to his pleasure because she feels less entitled to equal treatment with him (an interpersonal factor). Not having orgasms during partnered sex when one has orgasms during masturbation is unlikely to have a biological cause, so this one piece of the biopsychosocial puzzle is not likely to be relevant in Tamika's case. The importance of medical evaluations for possible biological influences on sexual functioning will be discussed later in the chapter. Age, health status, differing levels of ability, and other physical factors may be important in some cases. If, for example,

Tamika were suffering from multiple sclerosis (an autoimmune disorder that affects nerve cells), a change in her ability to experience orgasm may reflect a deterioration of her underlying disease state.

Sometimes patients will say that questions about sex are irrelevant as they are not currently, or have never been, in a relationship. To this I reply, "Okay, but you are still a sexual being." In addition to stimulating more exploration, this question is often enormously validating for people who have felt marginalized sexually by virtue of past experience, age, appearance, or other characteristics. Likewise, inquiry about masturbation also validates the patient's sexuality. When asking questions about masturbation, assume they do masturbate. The very few who do not will correct you. So instead of asking, "Do you masturbate?" ask instead, "How often do you masturbate?" or "Has the frequency of masturbation also changed since your divorce?" If the patient says, "Oh, I don't masturbate," ask, "Why not?" The answer is likely to be illuminating.

THE IMPORTANCE OF LANGUAGE

When discussing sex in psychotherapy, language is important. Patients may have a difficult time speaking honestly about sex. They often have very little practice doing so. Sometimes they stumble with language, unsure whether they need to know the proper medical terminology. They do not. Typically, I mirror the language my patients use. So in the imaginary dialogue with Tamika, when she said, "I don't cum," I used her words in my reply. If, however, a patient uses terminology I am uncomfortable with, I will instead use language that is more comfortable for me and hopefully acceptable to the patient. I avoid overly medicalized terminology, but sometimes it is helpful to bridge colloquial language that the patient uses with more formal terms to clarify meaning. If Tamika had said, "I don't get off when I have sex," I would have clarified her meaning: "Does that mean you don't have an orgasm when you have sex or that no aspect of it is pleasurable for you?" and also, "And by sex, do you mean any sexual activity, or are you talking specifically about intercourse?"

Often when I ask open-ended questions about sex, such as "Tell me about your first sexual experience" (a particularly useful question when exploring relationships and intimacy in assessment), patients will ask me to define sex. Heterosexuals wonder if I mean sexual intercourse. So, for all my patients, I usually leave the definition of sex up to them: "Tell me about your first sexual experience—however you define it." This revised question not only broadens the experiences I will hear about but also helps me to understand how the patient views sex: what counts as sex and what does not. This becomes important when couples are having conflicts about the frequency of sex, and one partner believes they just had sex while the other argues that it does not count for any number of reasons (there was no orgasm, it was not mutual, there was no penetration, it was too quick, or it was not enjoyable). It is also helpful when patients with a history of sexual abuse tell you that the abuse was their first sexual experience. George asked rather plaintively, "How do you think I feel knowing that my first sexual experience was with my mother?" which led to processing the importance of consent (his) in defining sex and unpacking the sense of blame and complicity he felt about the abuse.

Defining sex, what counts as sex, or what counts as important sexually can lead to surprising results. Consider the following case.

Sixteen-year-old Bridget was brought to therapy by her highly distraught mother. Bridget's mother had learned from one of her daughter's friends that Bridget had performed fellatio ("blow jobs" in her terminology) on 12 boys—all members of the school's basketball team—at a party the weekend prior. In session with me, Bridget described the event as "no big deal." I suspected that it was a big deal. None of her friends were talking to her, although they were talking about her. She was being ostracized and shamed. Because Bridget insisted it was no big deal and that "it wasn't really sex," we talked instead about her difficulties processing her friends' reactions and apparent abandonment. Many sessions later, when Bridget felt assured I was not shaming her, she began to open up about her sexual decision making the night of the party. None of her decisions were motivated by her own sexual desire or anticipation of her own pleasure. Bridget thought that giving blow jobs would make her popular, but as with many of her social decisions, she missed the mark. As we put the pieces of the puzzle together, the diagnosis of high-functioning autism spectrum disorder began to fit.

RESISTANCE

If patients do not want to talk about their sexuality, especially in the early sessions, it goes without saying that they do not have to. It is something you want to note, and important information if an otherwise open person says, "I don't want to talk about sex." Just for the record, in my 40 years of practice, no one has ever said that to me. In fact, one of my colleagues, upon returning to private practice after 20 years in an administrative position, remarked, "Everyone wants to talk about sex now!" It is true that many patients want to understand their sexuality, and it is a reasonable expectation that they will be open to therapeutic discussions that involve sex. There are, of course, exceptions. Had I pushed Bridget to talk about her sexual decisions early on in therapy, she likely would have shut down. Shame, as we will read in Chapter 4, is another reason a patient will find it difficult to talk about sex.

Some therapists ask for permission to talk about sex: "Is it okay if I ask you a few questions about sex?" I do not use this approach. In my opinion, it signals that there is something different and problematic about sex. We do not ask, "Is it okay if I ask you a few questions about the family you were raised in?" We just do it. And if our patients object—"I don't want to talk about my mother!"—we know there is work to be done.

IT IS NOT JUST WHAT THEY SAY BUT HOW THEY SAY IT

As therapists, we often notice how our patients speak about certain topics, and in psychotherapy we often ask our patients to stop and reflect. Assessment is more than the content of what people say. We take note of how our patients talk: their affect, language, body postures, and facial expressions. This helps us understand some of the deeper meanings attached to sex that our patients may not even be able to articulate. These include beliefs about their desirability or value, the meanings they attribute to their actions, and the very concept or idea they develop about their identity as a result of their sexual behaviors and the meanings ascribed. What we notice about how our patients talk about certain subjects is a critical part of the process of assessment and psychotherapy.

So in the case of Tamika, as we imagined a conversation about sex, there was a point where the therapist stopped and asked her to think about what she had just said—that she was not having good sex with a man she was uncertain she wanted to be with. This had therapeutic value for Tamika. But since Tamika's case is largely imaginary at this point, we can imagine a different scenario to highlight a metaexploration of her sexual concerns.

THERAPIST: You don't have orgasms with Bob? Is that unusual for you when you have sex with a partner?

TAMIKA: No. It's usually that way. Orgasms aren't that important really. I can enjoy sex without having an orgasm. It's the closeness I crave.

THERAPIST: What about your partners? Is that true for them too—that orgasms aren't important, that sex is about feeling close?

TAMIKA: (*laughs*) Oh, you're funny. No. Men need to cum. I mean, sex isn't really done until that happens. I would never just say, "Okay, I'm done" until he's had his orgasm.

THERAPIST: So, what do you think of that? That it's important for men to cum but not essential for you?

We can consider a number of possible responses from Tamika:

1. "I think it is really unfair, and I am not happy about it. I intend to make some changes."
2. "That's just the way it is. Men and women are different. It's biological. What are you going to do? You can't change Mother Nature."
3. "That's just the way it is. Men just really care only about getting off during sex. At least that's been my experience. Maybe I've never really been someone that men have cared about."
4. "It makes me feel strong to get my partner off—you know, actually it's power. I can get him to cum, but he can't do that for me."

How Tamika processes her orgasmic experiences (or lack thereof) provides more insight into the workings of her psyche. The potential responses included passive aggressiveness (4), helplessness (2), anger and an intention to make a change (1), and just another reflection that there is something about her that is inferior (3). Asking patients directly about their thoughts, beliefs, attitudes, and values as you ask them to reflect on their answers to your questions adds value to the assessment.

RESPECTING SEXUAL DIVERSITY

Patients are grateful not to be stereotyped, even if the stereotype fits. Do not make assumptions about your patient's sexual orientation, their gender identification, and their relationship constellations. Over the years, I have had this lesson reinforced many times. Not making assumptions about sex signals an openness to hearing anything the patient wants or needs to talk about in therapy. But especially for sexual minority patients, inquiry rather than assumption feels welcoming.

Recently, I met with Ellen, who had just moved to New Jersey from New York to take a job as a high school math teacher in one of the more prestigious private schools in the area. She arrived at her first session with me after work, so she was conservatively attired and well-groomed. She looked quite proper. Ellen had a history of depression and worried that her current loneliness might lead to another episode. Ellen reported that she was married. Many people would assume that Ellen was a cisgender heterosexual woman in a monogamous relationship. But she was not. My simply asking in our first session about other partners helped Ellen relax and trust me enough to open up about her life. (I simply asked, "Have you or your husband had any other sexual partners since your marriage?" Sometimes I ask, "What about other sexual partners?" even though I know the patient is married.) Ellen was in a polyamorous relationship—or open marriage, as she referred to it. Her loneliness was due to losing contact with her other partners when she relocated. Ellen had difficulty knowing whether she should negotiate new boundaries in her marriage. Could she ask her husband to spend more time with her? Did she even want to do that? And why was she having difficulty finding men who wanted to be in a part-time relationship? Was she not as attractive to men now that she was older? And what should she make of her growing attraction to women?

Asking about preferred pronouns on intake forms or in initial meetings can signal an openness to patients who are nonbinary. Asking "Are you currently in a relationship?" is preferable to inquiring about marital status. Asking about other sexual partners when working with an individual who is in a committed relationship invites disclosure of affairs as well as polyamory or consensual nonmonogamy. Asking about the gender of a current partner, even if it seems silly to do so, also signals openness. "Okay, so is it safe to assume that Robert is male? I'm guessing then that Tiffany is female? Do you have other sexual partners? Tell me about other significant relationships."

Although Ellen did not divulge her open marriage until asked, many patients who are members of a sexual minority group identify themselves as such at the intake. I am often asked if I have ever worked with people in polyamorous relationships, with nonbinary people, or with members of the kink community, and then, as a follow-up, whether this would be problematic for me. What might at first seem like a challenging or even hostile introduction is most often not. Ellen and others who have alternative sexual lifestyles have had their sexual choices blamed for their mental distress in ways that monogamous heterosexuals never encounter. If you have not worked with the sexual minority group in question, and you would like to work with the inquiring person, you can say something along the lines of, "I understand the need to ask this question, and while I haven't worked with others who [fill in the blank], I am open to doing so. I think you will find that I am a respectful and caring clinician, and I don't pathologize people's sexual choices." Just because Ellen did not want her polyamory to be blamed for her distress did not mean that polyamory was not a topic of therapy.

It was. It was because it was an important part of her life and the change in her polyamorous relationships was contributing to her depression. But her choice to be polyamorous was not pathologized.

Ellen talked about her difficulty feeling that she could be authentic in her relationships with new friends and colleagues for fear that they would be judgmental about her polyamory. We processed her difficulties with relationships ending and how this related to the loss of her partners in New York and her reticence to form new relationships. Ellen wanted to renegotiate some boundaries in her marriage, and we talked about her marriage. Had Ellen expressed unhappiness, distress, or concern about polyamory, we would have processed this in therapy (just as we would have had another patient felt uncomfortable in their monogamous lifestyle). But Ellen did not express discontent with her polyamorous orientation. Being polyamorous was an important and positive part of her identity.

RAISING THE TOPIC OF SEX IN ONGOING PSYCHOTHERAPY

Exploring sexuality in a thorough assessment requires the therapist to consider their patients as sexual beings. Sometimes this is more easily done at the beginning of therapy, before the intimacy of a strong therapeutic alliance makes an exploration of sexuality feel awkward and intrusive. This difficulty is addressed in many of the cases later in the book and more explicitly in Chapter 3 on "Ethical Boundaries." However, sometimes it can be rather obvious when the topic of sex is relevant. This brings us to Thomas.

Thomas is a cisgender, heterosexual, socially anxious young man with mild dysphoria. Although he wanted to be in a committed relationship, his dating relationships never went beyond a third meeting. This was despite the fact that he was attractive, well employed, and, in my estimation, a very nice person. I was certain that his social awkwardness was the problem, and we worked on his social skills as well as his negative core beliefs about himself. During one session Thomas was berating himself for his lack of social acumen: "It's like everyone else has the playbook and I don't." Although Thomas meant it as a sports analogy, his use of the word "playbook" slapped me in the face. I had not talked about sex with Thomas since our early sessions when he told me that he was not sexually active with anyone and had not been in a long while.

ME: Thomas, what does the playbook say about sex?

THOMAS: There's no sex in my playbook.

ME: Maybe that's part of the problem.

THOMAS: What? That no one wants to have sex with me?

ME: No, that part of your anxiety is that you don't know what to do about sex.

THOMAS: But I never get that far with anyone.

ME: Many of the dates you have and the women you meet, when you talk about them, I have no idea if you're attracted to them sexually or not.

This exchange led to a discussion of whether Thomas was aware of his sexual attractions; he was attracted from a distance, but on dates he froze and had no perception of his sexual feelings. We also discussed the notion of a sexual playbook and how he felt he lacked knowledge of what it was, as if there were one universal playbook (thank you, Masters and Johnson). The observation that Thomas was disconnected from his sexual feelings was an important one. Here is how we got to that:

ME: Tell me about the last time you had sex with a partner.

THOMAS: Oh. That would be with Gina.

ME: Gina? Gina was the girl you dated in university, right?

THOMAS: Junior year, yeah. We were set up by friends, but Gina was definitely the aggressor sexually, if we can say that.

ME: The aggressor?

THOMAS: We went out a couple of times, and then one night Gina kind of jumped me, if you know what I mean.

ME: Jumped you? Literally?

THOMAS: Pretty much. We were sitting around her room, and she just started taking off her clothes and kissing me and stuff.

ME: So she was pretty clear that she wanted to have some sort of sex with you.

THOMAS: No, she was clear she wanted to have sex. She basically got on top of me and told me she was on the pill.

ME: What was that like for you?

THOMAS: Great, actually. You know me. I would have dragged it out 'til forever.

ME: What was the sex like?

THOMAS: Pretty amazing, actually. I had never had sex before, and it felt fantastic.

ME: It felt fantastic because it was the first time?

THOMAS: It felt fantastic because I didn't have a chance to get nervous. She just took charge and made everything happen.

ME: So you didn't have to worry about anything (*Thomas nods yes*)—not about getting or keeping an erection and not about whether she wanted to have sex or not.

THOMAS: Exactly. I let her take charge.

ME: Tell me about the times you took charge.

THOMAS: (*embarrassed*) I never did.

ME: So letting Gina always take charge meant you didn't have to worry about what she wanted. And you didn't have to worry about whether you wanted to have sex or not, or what you might have wanted to do differently during sex.

THOMAS: Pretty much. Now that I think about it that way, I guess I'm waiting for someone else to take charge. Maybe they're waiting for me?

ME: So, what happened to end the relationship with Gina?

THOMAS: Well, she basically cheated on me with one of my roommates over the summer. She said I was boring.

ME: And what do you think—were you boring?

THOMAS: Yup. She was the first and only girl I had sex with. I never wanted to do anything wrong, you know—it was my first experience, and I wanted to get it right.

ME: So you wanted to get sex right. (*Thomas nods yes.*) And yet, Gina thought you were boring—not wrong, but boring.

As Thomas and I continued to work together, this exploration of his sexuality began to free him from his anxiety about "getting it right" and allowed him access to his sexual desires. This, in turn, helped Thomas not to be frozen on his dates. Noticing his own sexual attractions provided the motivation for Thomas to make the next move.

INTRODUCING SEX TO MOVE PSYCHOTHERAPY FORWARD

Having raised the topic of sex earlier with Thomas helped us to revisit it later in his therapy. It was helpful, but not essential. Discussing sex gave us a path forward and helped Thomas address his anxiety about dating. Discussing sex with Thomas moved his therapy forward as I hoped it would. Sometimes, as in the case of Tess and Dwight, raising the subject of sex may appear to be a bit of a last-ditch effort. There may not be an obvious reason to talk about sex, but there may not be other avenues of exploration open. In such cases, introducing the topic of sex could be a bit clumsy.

Tess and Dwight presented with a high degree of marital unhappiness primarily related to parenting issues. In their first session, Dwight, a reluctant participant in the therapy, talked about his love and admiration for Tess. Tess, a dynamic and successful marketing professional, was highly intelligent and strikingly beautiful. Tess had been born missing her lower left leg and, from adolescence on, made no effort with her clothing to hide or mask her prosthesis. In fact, she often decorated her prosthetic leg to highlight it. Tess agreed that having to contend with people's reactions to her leg and deal with multiple surgeries and fittings for her prosthesis, plus suffering the pain of several poorly fitting prosthetics, made her a "no bullshit, take me or leave me" person. Dwight, a meticulously dressed and bookish forensic accountant, had originally admired Tess's attitude, but this was now problematic for him.

The first few sessions I met with them were essentially the same: Tess complained about Dwight's inability to set limits with their children, and she cited numerous instances when he had undermined her authority with them. Dwight countered that she was too hard on the kids, set impossibly high standards, and would not listen to his input on rules before she set them.

It would not have been productive to rehash every parenting decision they were disputing, nor did I want to be a referee or a mediator. I wanted to understand why these two people could not negotiate reasonable compromises between them. So, I thought to ask about other areas of their lives that required negotiation, so yes, dear reader, I asked about sex. I interrupted one of their arguments and simply said, "It is hard for me to understand how the two of you can work well together on much of anything. Do you play well together? What about sex? What's your sex life like?" Although they were both a bit surprised by this sudden change of topic, they appeared to welcome it as well.

Tess and Dwight agreed that Tess was the sexual initiator; however, since the fighting began in earnest, the frequency of sex had decreased to about once a month, usually following a convivial evening out with friends. In individual sessions, the stories were clarified. Tess was tired of initiating sex, but she did want to have a sex life, and so when she was enjoying Dwight's company, she initiated sex. The sex was "good enough"; they both "got off," meaning that they each had orgasms. Their physiological responding was healthy, fine, and normal according to the Masters and Johnson (1966) model. It was just that there was no zing. Dwight gave much of the same story: good function, no flair. However, in his individual session and in response to my questions about what he wished sex could be, Dwight revealed that he wanted sex to be a bit kinkier than it currently was. He was specifically aroused by bondage and longed to tie Tess. Years ago he attempted to tie her with several of his neckties, but Tess told him that it reminded her of being restrained post-surgeries (so she would not tear at her dressings or disrupt the tubes going in and out of her body). She was sorry, but she just couldn't. This was a difficult issue, and yet another that they could not navigate together.

Sex was, however, an issue that inspired Dwight to more fully participate in therapy as he made the connection with how difficult he found it to engage as an equal with his formidable wife—both as a lover and as a coparent. Tess was also intrigued by the connection, and she was happy that Dwight was making more of an effort in therapy. Treatment focused on creating an equal partnership in all aspects of their lives but mainly focused on sex, decision making, and parenting. At the end of therapy, both Dwight and Tess were happy with how they were making decisions mutually regarding their children. They were also enjoying having sex again and were exploring how to play (sexually) with power, without the use of restraints.

Sometimes we reach a point in therapy when we feel stuck. The material being discussed is not being processed at a deeper level, and no behavioral changes are occurring. Being stuck can contribute to therapist burnout, and patients may drop out of therapy if the stalemate lasts too long. At times such as these, raising the topic of sex, or referring back to it if it was discussed earlier, can move therapy along. Once I understood Dwight's interest in bondage and Tess's negative reaction to restraints, I better understood the power dynamic at play, and I offered this perspective to them: "Power sharing seems to be difficult in your relationship, not only in parenting but also sexually. Tess, you never want to feel powerless, so you never 'give in' either to Dwight or even to your kids. Dwight, you are attracted to your strong wife, but you don't know how to interact with her, so you withdraw and just go along—in sex as in parenting." Tess and Dwight were intrigued by this interpretation, and I think they were as relieved as I was to have something else to focus on in terms of helping their relationship. Tess listened as Dwight talked about his interest in dominant–submissive sex play. Dwight listened as Tess related her reactions to his desires back to her feelings about power. This was the most listening they had done in months of therapy. The next week they came back having had sex and trying out some positions as directed by Dwight. Over the next several months of therapy, as their sex life improved, we were also able to work more effectively on their communication and "power sharing" regarding parenting and other domestic matters.

A synopsis of a complicated therapy (as most are) does not do justice to moments of sadness (as when Tess described her hospital stays) or levity (as Dwight recounted his neighbor marveling at his ability to tie knots) or frustrating times when their sexual encounters were disappointing and disconnecting. I do not mean to imply that raising the subject of sex will inevitably lead to treatment breakthroughs. It is important, if you bring up the subject of sex, not to just drop it. I asked Tess and Dwight about sex again the week after I first raised the subject: "So, last week we talked about sex. What were your reactions to that discussion?" This prompted Tess and Dwight to talk about the fact that they had had sex in the intervening time and that it was more enjoyable for each of them. "That's great. Tell me what was different." We did not necessarily talk about sex each session, but either they or I would often return to the subject. When the sex was disappointing (for example, when Tess began to criticize Dwight's choices and desires during sex), my response was not to take sides but to listen to their stories and helpfully commiserate with them: "I'm sorry to hear that. I can understand that each of you is disappointed in the outcome. What do you (to both Tess and Dwight) think is happening?" For example, I would be curious about whether Tess was reasserting her power or whether Dwight was withdrawing again.

REASONS FOR REFERRAL

When sexual material comes up in therapy, many psychotherapists believe that a specialist, a sex therapist, may be needed. In many ways, these clinicians are acting in what they believe to be their patients' best interests. But patients often feel they are being rejected because they brought up sex, or that the therapist is passing judgment, or now finds them less likable. In other words, you may feel that you are doing what is best, but your patients may not feel the same way. As you read through this book, I hope to highlight the skill set needed (and one you likely already possess) to address sexual problems in ongoing psychotherapy. Yet, there may be times to call in a specialist, either to consult or to take over the treatment. The following guidance might help.

You probably do not need to refer the patient to a specialist in the following cases:

- You are comfortable with the sexual content of the discussions in therapy. Or, even if the sexual material makes you feel uncomfortable, the patient is continuing to talk about the problem in therapy and finds talking with you helpful.
- You become more comfortable as the therapy progresses and so does the patient. You may have achieved this comfort by consulting trusted sources (books, websites, colleagues).
- You have checked with colleagues about your concerns regarding treatment, and they have reassured you. There seems to be little to no need for medical evaluation, as the patient is in good health.

In these instances, you should continue therapy with this patient. However, even when you continue therapy secure in the knowledge that you have the requisite skill set, it is best not to assume the role of expert. The rich diversity of human sexuality is such that no one person can be an expert on it all. Taking the role of expert also means distancing yourself from truly listening and understanding the sexual content of therapy. As you read through this book, you will find that the skills we already possess as therapists will allow us to treat most patients who are sexually confused, unhappy, or dissatisfied. I remind myself, with all my patients, that it is their sex life, not mine. Therefore, decisions about what to do sexually are their decisions to make, not mine to make for them.

You may need to refer the patient to a specialist in the following cases:

- Treatment progress seems to have reached a standstill.
- The patient is still distressed but is not finding it helpful to talk about sexual content in therapy.
- Your discomfort has increased or remains static.
- You feel frustrated with the lack of progress, or you feel helpless or incompetent.
- There are some sexual issues that the patient brings up that you do not understand, and these topics feel fundamentally different from other issues you have successfully addressed with this or other patients.

- Your colleagues do not know how to help.
- Medical issues may seem relevant, but you are not sure.

In these cases, you may want to consult with a sex therapist who can help you determine next steps (e.g., referral to a sexual medicine specialist or a referral to a sex therapist for a consult, or for ongoing treatment). If the medical issues seem important, you may want to refer the patient to a sexual medicine specialist. Some of these medical issues involve medication side effects, sexual pain, and erectile dysfunction (especially when the problem exists even during masturbation, or when nighttime erections cease, or any time that psychological variables do not seem to account for the problem). Do not refer a patient to a sex therapist without discussing the referral with the sex therapist first. You may find that you can continue to work with the patient, or you may decide together with the sex therapist to transfer the care of this patient to the sex therapist. One thing you should not do is refer the patient to a sex therapist to talk about sexual issues while you continue to see the patient for "all the other stuff." As you will discover as you read through this book, it is all connected and cannot be parsed or parceled out.

You need to refer the patient to someone else in the following cases:

- You do not feel that you can help the patient.
- You are uncomfortable with the sexual material being discussed, and that discomfort does not decrease with time, research, or consultation with colleagues.
- You find that you are judging the patient for their sexual thoughts and interests (and it is not clinical judgment but moral judgment).
- Treatment progress is stalled, and you have consulted with others to no avail.

The decision to refer may be difficult or not so difficult, and it may come as a relief or it may feel fraught. Please see Appendix D for a list of resources regarding sexual medicine and sex therapy consultants.

If you do refer, remember that the referral process is a collaborative one. The patient understands the reasons for the referral, even if they do not necessarily want to change therapists. When you have located an appropriate clinician and have discussed the case with them (with permission of the patient of course), you can talk further with the patient about the benefits of the referral while also processing their sense of loss regarding you. After the first or second visit with the new clinician, it will be helpful to reach out and see how the referral went. Many patients do not follow up on referrals unless they are guided through them.

Early in my career, when I was most unsure of myself, I was careless in making referrals. I thought patients would feel relieved to get a new therapist who would be more capable and competent than I. But after several therapists who took my referrals told me about how difficult the transition was for my former patients, I took notice. I now err on the side of being cautious and careful with referrals, taking the time in therapy to process the sense of loss patients may feel. I challenge myself to potentially suffer the embarrassment if a patient tells me, in so many words, that the referral is "no big deal." I at least want them to know that it is (and they are) a "big deal for me."

SUMMARY

Psychotherapy provides numerous opportunities to introduce and explore the subject of sex, including the initial evaluation, the ongoing process of therapy (when trust has been established), and when therapy appears to be stalled. When the therapist introduces a discussion of sex, it can convey an openness to explore sex and other sensitive topics, it can offer a path for therapeutic exploration, and it can provide a fresh direction for treatment. With some sensitivity to language and an awareness of the need for inclusivity, introducing discussions of sex into psychotherapy is within the skill set of psychotherapists. Nevertheless, there are several scenarios that might necessitate consultation or referral.

3 ETHICAL BOUNDARIES

Therapy is an inherently intimate process that requires firm boundaries, such as the assurance of confidentiality and the prohibition of dual relationships, including, and perhaps especially, sexual relationships between therapists and patients. Many therapists believe that avoiding the topic of sex altogether is an effective way of avoiding sexual feelings in therapy. I, of course, disagree. Sexual attractions do exist in psychotherapy, whether or not sex is explicitly discussed, and neglecting the topic of sex has risks, including the impoverishment of treatment outcomes.

This chapter addresses some ethical issues that may arise specifically when sex is a topic in psychotherapy. The main concern is usually that sexual boundaries will be crossed (or that, by talking about sex, a boundary will be loosened). This chapter outlines not only the pitfalls but also how to successfully avoid them so that discussions of sex can enhance treatment progress and outcomes.

https://doi.org/10.1037/0000483-004
Talking About Sex in Psychotherapy: A Guide for Every Therapist, by K. S. K. Hall

SEXUAL BOUNDARIES AND VIOLATIONS

The best statistics we have about the prevalence of sexual boundary violations is that approximately 10% of psychotherapists of varying professional disciplines have engaged in sexual contact with patients (Steinberg et al., 2021). This alarming statistic is based on therapist self-report and is therefore likely to be an underrepresentation of the prevalence of this problem. If you think this could never be you, you should consider that at one time, most of the therapists who have transgressed thought the same thing.

Sexual boundary violations include not only physical contact but also any sexualized or seductive interactions on the part of the therapist toward the patient. The difficult and tricky balance to strive for is well described thus:

> The challenge for all therapists in working in the heat of the powerful intimacy of speaking about sex is to find a psychological position that enables us to speak openly, directly and explicitly about this in a way that is reassuring and invites more openness while not being confusing or disturbing to the patient. (Goren, 2021, p. 130)

Sex therapists, who are trained to be comfortable with the subject of sex, are able to strike such a balance as they engage in the overt and clinically helpful discussions of sex that are the mainstay of their practice. The argument has been made that psychoanalysts may be less vulnerable to sexual malpractice because they are trained to be attuned to transference and countertransference issues and because they are also trained to note that "a cigar is not a cigar" (in other words, they are trained not to take sexual attractions as true or personal to them; Goren, 2021, p. 134).

The general consensus among clinicians and researchers who specialize in treating and studying sexual transgressions that occur in therapy is that sexual content in therapy is ignored at the therapist's peril and at the risk of patients' well-being. When sexual feelings and attractions arise in therapy, they need to be addressed. Ignoring a patient's sexual feelings may appear to be collusion or an implicit acknowledgment of a mutual attraction. Silence may allow a patient's fantasy to develop unchecked. Some therapists feel uncomfortable when they become aware of a patient's attraction to them and so assert boundaries in what often appears to the patient to be an overly restrictive and therefore punitive manner. It can be a difficult balancing act for a therapist if they too have intense (positive or negative) feelings about the patient and the patient's attraction to them. The risk is that therapists will err on the side of distancing from the patient; they may become overly rigid and objective in their manner such that the patient feels rejected and ashamed of their attraction (Goren, 2021).

Discussing a patient's sexual attraction can make most therapists feel uncomfortable, and it is important to be prepared for the possibility that one day you will have to have that conversation. Many years ago, I was working with a very socially anxious, very lonely, and very attractive man named Oliver. As we worked together, I began to wonder if Oliver had an attraction to me, or a secret wish that I would have a relationship with him and help him get over his anxiety. But it was only a feeling with no obvious evidence, so I tucked it away in the back of my mind. One day he reported the following dream:

> I am in an airplane, and the seat next to me is empty. The flight attendant comes by offering the usual—you know drinks, snacks. She has long, dark hair. She comes back and offers me more snacks. I am the only one she is offering seconds to, and that makes me feel special. Then she sits next to me and we talk. Pretty soon we are kissing and having sex right there in the seat! I know that all my problems are over, and I'm happy.

The one defining feature of the flight attendant was that she had long, dark hair. At the time, that described both the color and the style of my hair. I thought the dream provided an opportunity to discuss Oliver's secret wish to have sex with me: to discuss it, to understand it, and to help move Oliver forward in his therapy. But raising this topic made me feel vulnerable; I was not accustomed to being explicit about sexual attractions in therapy (or outside of therapy, for that matter!). When I told him what I thought the dream could be about, Oliver looked up at me in shock and said, no, the flight attendant was not me. Despite my interpretation that the plane represented the journey we were on together, the empty seat next to him signified his loneliness, the double snacks indicated he was special among all the passengers/my patients, and then the sex with the attendant/me was the answer, Oliver was surprised that I would even think that. I was internally mortified. Now what to do? "Will Oliver think I am attracted to him? Am I attracted to him? Was this all in my imagination?" I remained outwardly calm; I accepted Oliver's interpretation that the dream reflected only that he was a passive passenger in his life and that he needed an overt demonstration of interest in order to get over his anxiety and have a romantic and sexual relationship.

I do not have personal photographs in my office, and my professional listings do not have photos of me with family members or pets, or in exotic locations. I want my patients to know me intimately as a therapist, and to encounter me in the safe space of therapy. (Of course, some patients can and do snoop on the internet about their therapists—but those are boundary violations that can be discussed in therapy and are different from offering your patients a view of your happy family photos on your office wall.) As a rule, I do not touch or hug my patients. I do shake hands upon first meeting, and there are often hugs at the last meeting when therapy ends. I offer tissues when patients are crying. I look at them, I support them, I care about them. I am never, ever going to have sex with a patient, or former patient. These boundaries help me have confidence in my therapeutic approaches.

I was confident that I was not propositioning Oliver, which allowed me to ask him whether his dream was about a wish to have therapeutic sex. And Oliver agreed that it was; it just was not, according to him, a dream about therapeutic sex with me. It did lead us to a deeper discussion about his loneliness and what it would take for Oliver to have the confidence to have a relationship with a woman, including having sex. Perhaps I could have avoided my internal embarrassment by leaving myself out of my interpretation of his dream. But I think it was helpful for Oliver to know that I could consider that he was attracted to me and accept those feelings. I still do not quite believe that I was not the flight attendant in question, but that is my issue, not Oliver's.

I offer this example because too often we are taught to handle situations in which an aloof therapist is propositioned overtly by an unappealing patient. But therapy is an intimate process. And our patients are frequently appealing, lovable, and interesting. Part of what makes therapy work is that we often do love our patients, not romantically or sexually, but therapeutically. We see them in a way that they have yet to experience themselves, and for many patients their first experience of intimacy is in the safe space of therapy. Being a therapist is a position of power, but it is also a vulnerable position as we open ourselves up to caring for our patients.

SEXUAL ATTRACTION TO THE THERAPIST

When a patient has expressed sexual interest in me, I usually respond initially as I would to any compliment or expression of trust: "Thank you for trusting me enough to share your feelings with me." I often follow this up with a statement affirming the boundary: "I know you know that ethically, therapists cannot have any sort of dual relationship with their patients, including sexual relationships. I think this is a really important boundary." I would then go on to process the feeling of attraction in the context of the patient's presenting issues: "It's so rare that you trust someone enough to be vulnerable and open. I am thinking this means that those feelings of sexual desire that have eluded you in your relationships so far might be caught up in feelings of vulnerability that you protect yourself from experiencing."

If the patient asked, "Are you attracted to me?" I would answer, "I don't think of you as a potential sexual partner for me. You are my patient. But I am pretty certain that others would find you so. What do you think?"

Patients who are overt about having a sexual interest in their therapists, as are many patients with borderline personality disorder, do not represent the greatest challenge. I have had patients write me love letters, confess their strong sexual desires ("I can't even look at you, I want you so badly"), or tell me they have looked up the ethics code and mistakenly assume that "We can have sex 2 years after ending therapy, so let's end therapy now!" I have had patients who seemed to be aroused when discussing their sexual problems and others who seemed to have no boundaries: "Do you want to see my penis? I think it is too small; I need your opinion." Patients whose inappropriate behavior is clearly part of their larger psychopathology require intervention aimed at these larger issues; they need very firm boundaries, or sometimes, they need a different therapist. You cannot work with a patient if you feel intimidated or violated by them. But in my almost 40 years of doing therapy, inappropriate patients have been a tiny fraction of my practice.

When vulnerable patients encounter a caring, helpful therapist, it is not unusual for them to develop strong feelings, including sexual attraction, toward the therapist. Patients who have been sexually abused or those with low self-esteem may feel that their self-worth is tied to their sexual desirability. They may offer themselves sexually as a way to be more intimate or to ensure that the therapist will not abandon them. When sex is problematic, the patient may feel that sex with the therapist is the answer: "You understand me, you know all about me, you know all about sex. If I could have sex with you, that would help me." Typically, patients' sexual interest and even outright overtures are easy to resist, unless of course the therapist's mental health is vulnerable.

In my forensic work, I consulted on a case involving a sex therapist who had, in the course of his work, touched a patient on her breasts and vulva, underneath her clothing. He reported to me, "I felt drunk on power," because the patient idolized him at a time when his marriage was falling apart. The patient had come to see him because she felt sexually dead and believed that she could not respond to erotic touch. Over time, the patient came to believe that she would be responsive to the therapist's touch because he had brought her to life in many ways. The therapist was gratified by his patient's praise and desire. But instead of exploring what her attraction meant—was she now experiencing desire as a result of infatuation or his apparent unattainability? The therapist chose to believe that he did have the power to bring her to life. And so he touched her and brought her to orgasm in his office. After the session in which the touching occurred, the patient made a suicide attempt, unable to process what had happened and also believing that she had just cheated on her husband. Almost immediately remorseful, the therapist temporarily surrendered his license to practice and sought treatment. The Board of Psychological Examiners, which regulates the practice of psychology in the state, also required the temporary suspension, as well as treatment and a period of supervised and limited practice when the therapist returned to work.

It is this firm boundary of never having sex with our patients that makes the exploration of our patients' sexual thoughts, feelings, behaviors, and fantasies possible. Without that boundary, discussions of sex would be fraught with the idea that it might lead somewhere—it might lead to sex—and, of course, one would never know whose needs were actually being met.

The therapy relationship is an intimate one and can serve as a bridge to other intimate relationships, but it should not replace our patient's desire or need for other intimate connections. And our patients should not replace our need for intimate connections in our personal lives. Mentally and emotionally vulnerable therapists may cross the line that separates compassion from abuse. It is incumbent upon us, in our role as therapists, to look after our own mental health and to understand the challenges of working with patients who may imbue us with exceptional qualities that, in other circumstances, would be extraordinarily gratifying.

Ongoing supervision, being in your own therapy, attending conferences, reading the literature on therapy and ethics, and having trusted colleagues you can turn to are all helpful antidotes to the vulnerabilities that precede boundary violations by therapists. The two most important things we can do as therapists to avoid crossing sexual boundaries and hurting our patients are to take care of our own mental health and to work on becoming more comfortable talking about sex in psychotherapy.

SEXUAL ATTRACTION TO PATIENTS

It is important to acknowledge that there is an inherent power imbalance in psychotherapy: There is a patient who needs help and a knowledgeable therapist who has the expertise (power) to help. When a therapist is attracted to a patient, it is good practice for the therapist to discuss their feelings with a colleague, but not to share them with the patient. Good boundaries require an awareness of what is our own issue as a therapist and a person and what is therapeutically relevant for our patients. Even when you are confident that you will not act, sexual attraction to patients can impair the therapy. It can lead to avoiding the topic of sex altogether, thereby prematurely eliminating an avenue of psychotherapeutic exploration or denying a patient needed help regarding sexual concerns, or it may lead to overly rosy assumptions about a patient's functioning. It can limit our trust in our own therapeutic judgment. An attraction to a patient may also lead us to initiate or prolong discussions of their sex life, far past what is therapeutically helpful. Consider the case of Susanne, whose therapist confessed his love for her.

Susanne, herself a psychotherapist, came to see me due to depression. She felt profoundly ashamed of having had a sexual relationship with her previous therapist, Dr. L. Ironically, Susanne went to see Dr. L after a devastating end to an affair in which her affair partner chose to stay with his wife. In this vulnerable state of feeling rejected but not entitled to feel that way, and not wanting to risk future rejection, Susanne was a very gratifying patient. She never missed an appointment, paid promptly, invariably flattered Dr. L by recalling something extremely helpful from the previous session, and made an effort to dress well for her sessions, never wearing the same outfit twice. Dr. L, hoping to improve Susanne's self-esteem, would often comment on how nice Susanne looked, what a lovely color for her, and so forth. But instead of building her confidence, he created an anxious pattern where Susanne felt that she had to look good for Dr. L. She became increasingly reliant on his opinion of her, and soon she was bringing him gifts, flattering him as a skilled therapist, and expressing interest in him (asking about his health, his family). They had an affair for almost 3 years, despite the fact that Susanne admitted she never really enjoyed sex with Dr. L and had never wanted to have an affair with him. But when he told her that he was falling in love with her, and when he initiated sex by placing his hand on her knee and kissing her, she felt she could not say no. Had Dr. L not been gratified by Susanne's attentions, he could instead have noticed aloud, "It seems like you are putting a lot of pressure on yourself to be a good patient for me." He could have gently challenged her: "You don't need to do all that for me to want to work with you."

Disclosing attraction to a patient is usually the end of a string of inappropriate disclosures on the part of the therapist. Therapist self-disclosure, when genuine and in the moment, is considered an important therapeutic tool according to some schools of therapy (e.g., existential, feminist, relational psychotherapies). But sexual abuse of patients often starts with therapists sharing intimate details of their own lives (often under the guise of communicating understanding and empathy). Sometimes this sharing includes disclosing feelings of loneliness, marital unhappiness, or lack of sexual fulfillment. Patients have discussed the confusing revelation of a therapist's attraction and how this constrains therapy and often makes the patient feel obligated to engage sexually (as Susanne did). Therapists who practice self-disclosure should have a boundary for discussing sexual attraction. Therapists not accustomed to self-disclosure should know never to discuss their sexual attractions. Without having self-disclosure grounded in therapeutic philosophy and technique, and without training and supervision in self-disclosure, disclosing a sexual attraction is very likely to be self-serving.

Susanne never told Dr. L that she did not enjoy having a sexual relationship with him. Although he stopped charging her for sessions, the time allotted for her therapy was instead used for the two of them to have sex. Without therapy, and finding herself again having an extramarital affair, Susanne somehow found the strength to end her relationship with Dr. L. For years afterward, Dr. L sent Susanne emails and texts telling her he missed her and that she was the love of his life. Susanne feels a combination of anger and protectiveness toward Dr. L and shame about her involvement with him. She is adamant that she will never file a complaint against him. This is not unusual; most patients do not report therapist abuse. Respecting her autonomy in decision making and maintaining her confidentiality superseded my option of reporting Dr. L's unethical behavior (Bailey & Brown, 2021).

A final caveat about therapist self-disclosure involves patients' requests for recommendations regarding sex toys, websites, apps, books, or movies about sex that could provide erotic inspiration for the patient. While often innocuous, there is the possibility for the therapist to reveal too much about their own sexual preferences or to overly influence the patients' choices (perhaps the therapist only provides access to straight porn for a bisexual patient or recommends a dildo instead of a clitoral stimulator as the vibrator of choice). Instead, I help patients learn to navigate the often-confusing array of options. I suggest that they read reviews of books on the bookseller's or publisher's website to get an idea of the possible appeal of a book, and I caution them about pop-up advertisements on porn sites and encourage them to do a bit of their own research on the sites before subscribing or doing too much exploration. I will encourage them to use their judgment about online stores and privacy and security. Patients usually appreciate the fact that while I do not suggest certain sites or apps, I am available to discuss with them what they discover, as well as their concerns and delights, as they navigate this terrain.

HARMING THE PROFESSION

Crossing sexual boundaries in psychotherapy harms not only the patient but also the profession and practice of psychotherapy. Psychotherapy is built upon trust; as that trust erodes, so does the effectiveness of our practice. Back in the early days of sex therapy, when many people were confused about what exactly sex therapy was, I would start therapy by explaining that sex therapy was talk therapy and that while there might be homework exercises for the patient to do on their own at home, there would never be any sexual contact with the therapist, or anything sexual happening in the office. I have not felt the need to be that explicit for many years. But if trust in our professional ethics erodes, I may reconsider. We specify other procedures when we begin therapy with a new patient, such as cancellation policies and confidentiality, so a discussion of sexual boundaries is not out of line.

DISTINGUISHING EXPLOITATION FROM THERAPEUTIC EXPLORATION

A comprehensive approach to psychotherapy will necessarily involve some discussions about sex. One important distinction we need to make when understanding the sexual difficulties our patients are experiencing is this: Is the sexual problem due to the quality of sex, is the problem reflective of underlying psychological issues, or both? In these situations, we need to ask detailed questions about their sexual activities. With one last look at Tamika's lack of orgasms with a new boyfriend, the question arose as to whether he was a skilled lover. In other words, a therapist might need to ask Tamika what kind of sexual stimulation she was receiving when she was having orgasm-less sex. Asking about her thoughts, feelings, physical sensations, and activities (e.g., Is there clitoral stimulation?) would be part of the process of helping Tamika understand her own sexual responses. But this is tricky. Explicit discussions of what our patients are doing sexually bring us dangerously close to sexualizing them. Where is the line separating exploitation from therapeutic exploration?

Sex is highly personal. There are no scales that measure the right amount of stimulation needed for orgasm, or for erections or vaginal lubrication. There is a great deal of variation in what people find arousing and in what amount. This means that we often have to use our judgment as to whether there is sufficient stimulation for sexual responding to occur. In fact, the *Diagnostic and Statistical Manual of Mental Disorders* (5th ed.; *DSM-5*; American Psychiatric Association, 2013; as well as earlier editions) tasks us with this determination. For example, regarding the diagnosis of female orgasmic disorder, the *DSM-5* states, "It is also important to consider whether orgasmic difficulties are the result of inadequate sexual stimulation; in these cases, there may still be a need for care, but a diagnosis of female orgasmic disorder would not be made"

(American Psychiatric Association, 2013, p. 430). The extreme ends of the spectrum (too little, more than enough) are always easier to deduce than the murky middle.

My hairdresser asked me years ago for some advice about an orgasm cream she was considering adding to the line of personal products at her salon. The title on the marketing package she received proclaimed that "10,000 screaming women can't be wrong." The product claimed to help women have orgasms during partnered sex. As far as I could tell from the list of ingredients, this seemed to be a concoction primarily containing menthol, a natural derivative from spearmint or peppermint that leaves a cooling sensation when applied to the skin. The instructions directed the woman's partner to apply the product to her clitoris during foreplay and rub for 10 minutes, applying more of the ointment as necessary and desired while following the woman's directions as to the pressure and speed of the rubbing. I was pretty certain that in most situations, this would be sufficient stimulation for an orgasm to occur. I was also pretty certain that the menthol ointment was beside the point.

Luckily, when working with sexual issues, it is really the patient who must be the expert. Recall that arousal and desire often work in a feedback loop, according to Basson's (2001) circular model. So, if there is sufficient arousal, there should also be a desire for more, and the desire for more should help the person get more stimulation, further increasing arousal, until the point of orgasm. A helpful mode of inquiry is one that would help patients and therapists understand what might be interfering with this cycle while also letting the patients be the experts on their own sexual desires and responses. Questions might include "Did you feel that you wanted her to keep touching your breasts before moving on to oral sex?"; "Might those anxious thoughts explain why you felt ticklish when she went down on you (cunnilingus)?"; and "What stopped you from asking for some anal stimulation when that is what your body was craving?" From this sexually explicit discussion with a patient, you might find out not only whether there was sufficient stimulation needed for her arousal and orgasm but also how (dis)connected she is to her body, how she communicates (or does not) with a partner, and how much stress she puts on herself to please another, sometimes at the cost of her own needs, wants, and pleasure. But this brief discussion may also feel dangerously close to an intrusive or seductive exchange with a patient.

What separates exploitation from therapeutic exploration is the reason behind the questions. If the motivation is to understand what is interfering with the feedback loop of arousal and desire, then the questions are necessary, helpful, and appropriate. It is exploitative to simply be curious or to derive or seek sexual gratification from sexually explicit discussions (and the images they may evoke in your mind). Your comfort in asking these questions, built partly on your confidence in the reason you are asking, is also key to communicating to the patient that this is therapy, not personal interest.

The story of my therapy with Luis illustrates the tricky balancing act and the therapeutic value of talking about sex in psychotherapy. I provide a lot of detail in this case so you can see the intimacy of the therapy and understand the choices that need to be made while remaining aware of the importance of boundaries.

Luis was reminiscent of a cubist painting by Pablo Picasso. Composed of many parts that should not really go together, he had a startling and pleasing appearance. His crooked (once broken) nose, large eyes, small mouth, and disappearing jaw formed a rather mesmerizing face. His mother was Puerto Rican; his father, Irish. His background was one of working-class poverty, but he was currently in the upper edges of middle class. He had not gone to college but was extraordinarily well-read; he exuded confidence but was anxious and depressed. Luis was a hardworking man for whom nothing came easy. He put me on notice right away that his therapy would also not be easy. He had an intensity that made me realize Luis was going to need and want the best of me. I liked that challenge.

Luis came to see me after a series of relationships had ended badly. These endings had left Luis in despair. "I can always kill myself," he told me in our first meeting when he talked about not having any hope for a lasting, meaningful connection. Luis was not suicidal; he very much wanted to live. But he did not know if his life would ever involve the intimate relationship he craved. Still, there was a violence in the way he talked about his emotions. It had the effect of keeping me away when I also knew he was telling me about his desperate need to be close. It took emotional energy to stay present with Luis.

"I can always tell when a woman is about to end it with me," he said one session several months into our therapy. "I can tell because I start having problems with sex." When I had asked Luis in earlier sessions about sex, he had failed to mention this important point. "That's interesting," I said. "Can you tell me more about this ability you have?" Over the next several sessions, as Luis talked about his erection problems being the early warning signal for a relationship in distress—his canary in a coal mine, if you will—I was piecing together a very compelling picture of a very complicated man. Over the course of our therapy, Luis's story often broke my heart, while his courage and vulnerability led me to feel love for him.

Luis was raised in poverty, in a violent neighborhood, and in a violent home. His father (now deceased) was mostly silent and sat at home staring into space or blankly watching television. But then sometimes, and inexplicably, he would fly into fits of rage, beating his wife and children. Luis's father was unemployed, while his mother worked as a cleaner in the apartment building in which they lived. Both of these factors were sources of great embarrassment for Luis. Largely neglected, Luis and his sister, 2 years his senior, were left to navigate life on their own. When they were in their early teens, his sister had a reputation for being sexually "easy," which was another source of shame for Luis. At school, he tried to keep his head high and act as though nothing bothered him, but in reality, he spent his evenings looking for his sister to make sure she was safe and would often bring her home after a date that ended badly. Luis was fiercely loyal to his sister and got into several fights at school defending her reputation (hence Luis's broken nose). Luis did not date in high school, fearing that no one would want to go out with him and knowing he did not have the money to pay for the ordinary things people did on dates. The money Luis made from his paper routes and after-school jobs went to keeping the electricity on in the apartment or putting groceries on the table. When Luis graduated from high school, he immediately went to work, starting as a stock room clerk in a furniture store and working his way up, as per the American dream, to become a buyer for the furniture franchise. Once he had a bit of money, Luis began to curate his life. Everything had to look a certain way; there could be no reflection of his shameful and impoverished background.

I had no doubt that Luis could sense when things were about to go badly in a relationship. After years of vigilance, watching for any small sign of his father's impending rage, Luis had likely become attuned to subtle signals of dissatisfaction that would likely trigger anxiety. So, this is what happened as Luis and I explored his sexual difficulties:

ME: Luis, you said that you can tell that there are problems in the relationship because you start to have difficulty getting an erection. Can you tell me more about that?

LUIS: (*rolling his eyes*) What do you want me to say? I already told you that I have trouble getting hard. Isn't that embarrassing enough?

ME: I get it. It is embarrassing to experience that and embarrassing to have to relive it by talking about it with me. But I need to understand what is happening in order to help.

LUIS: No, I know. I get it. It's just embarrassing.

(He gets up and paces back and forth before walking toward the window in my office. I have a brief moment of worry that he will jump out. But like many people with anxiety, it helps Luis to see an exit, no matter how unlikely it is, and after a moment he sits back down.)

ME: Tell me about the last time this happened, when you didn't get an erection. (Situating the question in a particular context is often more helpful than asking about generalities.)

LUIS: (*taking a deep breath*) Lily and I were at my place. I made a nice dinner, I mean really nice. (He describes the meal; it sounded delicious.) After dinner we were sitting on the couch and having drinks. We were kissing, and she was giving me all the signals that she wanted to have sex. But nothing was happening for me.

ME: You noticed that you were not getting sexually aroused? (*Luis nods.*) You weren't getting an erection, or at least enough of an erection?

LUIS: Nothing! Dead! Oh, God, do we have to talk about this?

ME: What about the rest of your body? What was happening there?

LUIS: My heart was racing, and I was starting to sweat a bit, at least I think I was starting to sweat. I was getting hot. I was panicking.

ME: What was going on in your head?

LUIS: Ah, my head. A million things at once. I was thinking I should be getting hard, but I'm not. I was thinking I'm a loser. I was thinking, weirdly, about the fact that Lily didn't eat the scalloped potatoes I made. I was thinking she is going to leave me if I can't get it up. I was thinking it's a disaster.

ME: Wow, that is a lot. But I think you have some unrealistic expectations about your sexual functioning. I mean, maybe you just needed some physical stimulation in order to get hard?

LUIS: Oh, my God. You really don't get it. I should not have to have her touch me in order to get an erection. That is so pathetic. I shouldn't need that. She's a beautiful woman who wants to have sex, and I need more than that? That is pathetic.

ME: Actually, it's not pathetic. It may just be what you needed in the moment.

LUIS: I just want sex to be easy. You know? I just want to have an erection when we take our clothes off. I don't want my girlfriend to have to help me with that. I just don't.

ME: It would be nice, for sex to be easy. But maybe what you're envisioning as pathetic wouldn't actually be so difficult. You know, for Lily to touch you, to arouse you.

LUIS: She'll think I'm pathetic.

ME: Maybe she would enjoy turning you on?

LUIS: (*long pause*) Would you? I mean, is this just hypothetical bullshit or what? (He is staring at me intensely, and I can feel the tension inside him. He is not angry. He is desperate and pleading. I know there are only seconds to answer before he can no longer contain his emotions, before he gets up and leaves.)

ME: (I'm a bit panicked. This is a big ask and extremely vulnerable for Luis. I'm thinking, "Don't screw this up.") Luis, you're asking if I—personally—would enjoy arousing you? And I guess you're thinking if the answer is yes, then maybe you can believe me, that you are not pathetic. But that answer would be the hypothetical you are dismissing. I'm your therapist. I can't ever engage with you sexually. So, you are still faced with the problem that it is really hard to believe that a woman would enjoy giving you sexual pleasure. And so it's hard to be vulnerable.

LUIS: Oh, God, I'm sorry. I'm sorry. I shouldn't have said that. I'm so fucking pathetic. Are we okay?

ME: Luis, we are okay. I'm touched that you asked me that question. It is so hard for you to be vulnerable, and you were in that moment. But that is a lot of power you would be giving me, or any woman, to determine whether or not you are pathetic.

LUIS: I feel like jumping off a bridge.

ME: You feel like jumping off a bridge?

LUIS: I feel so awful. I want to leave.

ME: Thank you for trusting me Luis. Thank you for trusting me enough to talk about this issue.

LUIS: (*angrily*) It's not an "issue." It's a monumental disaster.

ME: A monumental disaster.

LUIS: (*insistently*) For me, a monumental disaster for me. I can't bear it.

ME: I understand. You have worked so hard to be where you are, to be successful. And yet hard work cannot help you get an erection.

LUIS: (*agitated*) Well, what will? What?

ME: Being turned on. Feeling aroused.

LUIS: (*incredulous*) Oh, my God! Really? I'm with beautiful women; if that doesn't do it . . . I'm hopeless.

ME: You're right. Beautiful women are not enough. This is not just about your brain thinking "She's beautiful"; it's about experiencing it in your body.

LUIS: I hate my body.

This led us to a discussion of his disgust with his appearance, which related to his fear of being like his father (he looked like him). As we talked about the fear of being like his father, we began to process his fear of his father. Noticing the scalloped potatoes that were left uneaten (and that neither Luis nor Lily talked about) triggered Luis's anxiety about impending trouble. This anxiety was too intense to be just about the potatoes and was likely a post-traumatic response. This intense anxiety interfered with his ability to get an erection, which triggered even more anxiety.

Over the course of our therapy, Luis brought me several small gifts: a Freud finger puppet, tomatoes from his garden, and cocktail napkins with jokes about therapy (Hostess: So, are you seeing someone? Me: You mean like a therapist? Or a hallucination?). I did not refuse or interpret these gifts. Were they boundary violations? Not to me. I knew that little by little, Luis was offering me small pieces of himself, and I was not about to reject him. Apart from these tokens, he never crossed a line—the gifts were never extravagant or overly personal, he never lingered to extend the time of the session, and he did not call between sessions unless he was in crisis (which happened once). Luis came to trust me inside the safe boundaries of therapy. These same firm boundaries became even more important and necessary as we explored what was so difficult and painful for Luis to consider: his desire.

And this is where exploring his sexual fantasies became helpful.

SEXUAL FANTASIES

Sometimes people, like Luis, have a difficult time knowing or conveying what they desire sexually. It is often conflated with what they think they should desire, based on the cultural landscape in which they find themselves. Luis did not want to replay a sexual script based on the machismo culture of his neighborhood, a culture that badly treated his sister. He relied instead on his interpretation of romance from what he gleaned from the larger Western culture in which he lived. Every relationship was the same; he spent a lot of time and money curating his dates: flowers, dinners, romantic walks, him wearing just the right clothing, and her, hopefully, looking beautiful. Sex would happen quickly in these relationships (first or second date), and Luis followed the same sexual script each time (remove her clothing, admire her body, remove his own clothing to reveal an erection, caress her and stimulate her to orgasm, have intercourse, ejaculate, and lie in each other's arms). This rigid sexual script served to keep anxiety at bay. Luis would find it difficult to keep his erection should his partner deviate from the script: She didn't have an orgasm! She brought a vibrator! She wanted to have quick sex! She looked bored! She didn't like the scalloped potatoes! Luis was appalled when I suggested that he might need some physical stimulation from his partner to get or maintain an erection ("Maybe you need her to touch you—caress your penis or put her mouth on your penis"). Just the idea of not presenting his partner with his erect penis agitated Luis and made him feel much too vulnerable. It was difficult to explore his desires in the context of his past and current sexual relationships. So, I asked him about his sexual fantasies.

Sexual fantasies are extremely private and personal, and the reason to explore fantasies with patients is that other ways of accessing their desire have not yielded results. In a way that is similar to sexual dreams (remember Oliver), sexual fantasies can sometimes be about sexual desire for the therapist. One should always approach the exploration of sexual wishes and fantasies with this possibility in mind and with strict boundaries as the guardrails. No matter how gratifying you might find it to be the object of your patient's desire, remember, it is really not about you; it is about the idealized you, the therapist you. Patients sometime say, "I wish we could be friends." In a way this is an acknowledgment of the fact that they are comfortable in therapy, that they like me (insofar as they know me), and that they are curious about what a relationship with me would be like outside of therapy. If it is true, I might reply that if we met somewhere other than therapy, we might have become friends. But in my head, I know that at least part of what is compelling about being friends with me is actually what is so wonderful about therapy: a time when another interesting person is interested and focused solely and completely on you. So, when a patient says they fantasize about you, it is the therapist you, the idealized person who is steady, steadfast, helpful, interested, and focused on them, that is the object of desire. It is not the you who expects a lot from your partner, who is often easily irritated, who is grouchy before your morning coffee, who is distracted by their phone during dinner, and who does not look so good in the morning—not that you.

I asked Luis directly about what he desired. He gave me the usual—what he was doing was what he desired. I asked Luis if there were any books or stories that he found erotic, and he answered that he did not read fiction. I asked him about movies or shows he had watched that he might have found erotic, at least in part. Luis replied that he did not want to be like his father, spaced out in front of a screen, ergo, he did not watch shows and he did not watch porn. When I asked Luis directly about the content of his sexual fantasies ("What do you think about when you masturbate? What images come into your mind as you are pleasuring yourself?"), at first he gave me his standard fare from his usual sexual script. This of course I accepted, but then I also probed more: "Are there some sexual fantasies you have that perhaps you wish you didn't have, or ones that you don't understand? Any recurrent sexual fantasies?" With this last question, Luis rather sheepishly told me that he does have a recurring fantasy. In this fantasy, a neighbor knocks on his door and wants to borrow a cup of sugar for some baking she is doing. Although he is still sweaty from his workout, he leads her to the kitchen. He can feel the sexual tension. He reaches over her to get the sugar from the cabinet and brushes against her. The sparks fly, and she is kissing him, taking off his clothes, and they have mind-blowing, passionate sex on the kitchen floor.

ME: That is such a rich fantasy.

LUIS: Really? I think it's lame—Tarzan meets a 1950s housewife.

ME: It is a rich fantasy because it so strongly conveys how very much you want to be desired, for just being you. (Luis begins to tear up, then composes himself. He looks at me expectantly, but I let the silence stay.)

LUIS: It's never going to happen.

ME: What?

LUIS: Desire like that, for me. It's never happened. I've always had to make everything perfect to even convince a woman to come home with me.

ME: Luis, I won't argue with you, although I strongly suspect you're wrong. I think that you orchestrate everything because you are too anxious to see if there is desire there for you, without all the trimmings.

Over the course of a little more than a year, I worked with Luis on several fronts. We processed the trauma of his father's physical abuse and rages. We talked through his shame related to sex, his sister, and his unrequited sexual desires during adolescence. He explored his anger and sadness and guilt related to his mother, who he felt abandoned him, but whose hard work had provided the family with a home. We talked about his loneliness and his desire for a lasting connection. When we approached the midpoint of the second year of therapy, we came to more fully appreciate the fact that his sexual desires mirrored his longing to be part of a traditional relationship. His sexual fantasy mirrored his wish to be accepted for who he is (Tarzan, the boy raised in the jungle).

With the foundation of a solid therapeutic relationship, Luis trusted me to help him navigate the world in a new way, and we came up with a plan to move forward. Essentially, Luis agreed to slow down, to try to allow some space for women to express interest in him. Luis needed help reading that interest, however, and he would often ask me what certain things meant: "A woman sent me a text message with kisses at the end—what does that mean? A woman I just met asked to meet for coffee—is that a date? A woman I used to work with sent me a card thanking me for being a good colleague—what should I say?" My answer was usually the same: "What do you think/feel/want to do?"

After many months, Luis was dating again. He was practicing slowing things down so that he could process his feelings in real time: "Am I attracted to her? What types of sexual things am I wanting (from kissing and touching to more overt sexual behaviors such as oral sex and intercourse)? Do I feel that she is attracted to me (as opposed to a worry that she is likely not attracted to him)? How does it feel when she touches me? How does it feel when I touch her?" The feelings that Luis processed were both emotional and sensual. I would ask Luis to focus on the sensual elements of touch: softness, warmth, smoothness, and tingling sensations. Luis was initially very reluctant to slow things down sexually, worried that the women he was dating would be disappointed. But he found, to his surprise, that most of the women were very happy to go at a pace that was comfortable for him.

Luis told me many times how much he valued the fact that I was steady and supportive, and that I was not giving up on him. After 3 years of therapy, Luis told me he had fallen in love. When he gave me the details, I thought to myself, "This will be a disaster." He met Phoebe through friends from his old neighborhood. She was a recovering heroin addict and had been clean for about 6 months. I was protective of Luis and urged caution but did not go further than that (I rarely, if ever, tell patients to end a relationship, and I never tell a patient to commit to someone; it is their life and their choice). Luis took my cautionary words as a sign that I cared about him (which was true). But he pursued a relationship with Phoebe (the woman in question). He took it slow and implemented many of the strategies for centering on his feelings, both emotional and sensual, as we had discussed. He was very attracted to her. And he enjoyed taking care of her, sometimes going with her to her Narcotics Anonymous meetings and also attending Al-Anon meetings on his own.[1] His skill set in curating his environment helped them build a life of sobriety together. Despite my initial skepticism, they are still together, a fact I know from the yearly cards I still receive from Luis. Luis delights in the knowledge that I was wrong about Phoebe. It made him realize that he could trust his own judgment.

In our last session Luis asked me if it was all right if he told me he loved me. He added that I need not tell him my feelings, although he said he was pretty sure I cared a lot about him. Luis said that it was his feeling that I truly cared about him that allowed him to take the risks he took in therapy. He said he would never have talked about his sexual fears had he not been certain I cared about him. I did tell Luis that I cared deeply about him and that, over our time together, I had grown to love him. We agreed that he could and would send me periodic updates about his life. And with that, Luis left therapy ready to risk a relationship with Phoebe.

IATROGENIC HARM AND THE RUSH TO REASSURE

Iatrogenic harm in psychotherapy refers to harm that occurs as a result of a therapist's actions or that result from a misapplication of the therapy itself. Having sex with a patient is clearly one form of harm. But there are others, specifically that in our rush to reassure our patients, or to calm or assuage them, we unwittingly prevent them from doing the hard work of therapy. Our own discomfort may likewise propel us to be reassuring rather than therapeutic, leading us to prematurely cut off conversations about sexuality. We can look back at several decision points in Luis's therapy to understand how I managed to stay out of trouble and how my interventions served to help rather than harm Luis.

Luis's need for connection was great; his emotions were intense, and his ability to calm himself was poor. This was a difficult combination. Luis often paced the room, ran his fingers through his hair, spoke of wanting to jump off a bridge, and occasionally seemed to be in physical pain. Because I cared about Luis, it was hard to see him in agony. I wanted to circumvent the hard parts of therapy for him and reassure him that it would be all right.

The first decision point between reassurance and deeper exploration was when Luis asked me, in desperation, whether if I were his sexual partner,

[1]Al-Anon is a group support program that originated as an outgrowth of Alcoholics Anonymous to help family members cope with a loved one's drinking. Many people find the support helpful in coping with a loved one's addiction to drugs as well.

I would enjoy stimulating him to erection. In haste and feeling pressured, I could certainly see the possibility of wanting to reassure Luis, to calm him down, and to convey to him that he is not repulsive. The intensity of his ask combined with the follow-up question of whether "this is just hypothetical bullshit" put me on the defensive. So, if I wanted to calm him, I might have said something like "This is not hypothetical bullshit. I care about you. And if I were your sexual partner, I would very much enjoy turning you on." If I had said that, or something like it, I would have taken a step closer to the edge of the slippery slope of crossing a sexual boundary. But even if that boundary was not ever crossed, that reassuring answer might have served only to gain some fleeting calm. It would have been confusing to Luis. It likely would have provoked further turmoil because, over time and in an anxious person's mind, all sorts of scenarios can be in play: "Should I have sex with my therapist? Does she want to have sex with me? What should I do? Will she be upset if I have sex with other women?" Our patients may be prone to idealize us at some point in therapy. We do not need to encourage this by setting ourselves up as an ideal partner who can never be had: "Of course, I would want to stimulate you. These other women are not as generous as I am. It's too bad we can't be together."

By the way, stepping close to the edge, but not falling down the slippery slope, leaves open the option of stepping back to safety. If I had said something inappropriate, I might still be able to salvage the therapy. In the next session, I could have said something like this:

> Luis, I was thinking about our discussion in the last session, and my answer to one of your questions was that I wouldn't reject you if you didn't have an erection, and that I would enjoy turning you on. I thought about that, and I had no right to answer you in that way, and I'm sorry. I don't think of you in a sexual way; you're my patient. So it was the hypothetical bullshit you called me on. What I should have done is encouraged you to explore why you think you must have an erection to present to a woman. I would want to explore that with you. Maybe we could do that now?

The second decision point was accepting Luis's gifts. My interpretation of his gifting was that he was giving me parts of himself, that he felt so grateful to me for caring about him, and that he wanted to express it by giving me these tokens of appreciation. It was a big risk for Luis. I felt that I would have hurt him very badly if I had said, "Thank you, Luis. Unfortunately, ethically therapists are not supposed to accept gifts from their patients." Or if I had interpreted the meaning of his gift: "I wonder if your gifts mean that you think about me when you are not in session, and if by giving me these small tokens, you are hoping that I will think about you when we are not together as well." I had to trust my judgment that these were expressions of gratitude and extensions of himself that meant that Luis was trusting me. It would have been different if Luis had gifted me tickets to the World Cup or to a sold-out Broadway show—expensive, valuable gifts that I would want to accept but would have to say no. Those gifts would have a different meaning, likely that Luis would feel he had to buy my interest and attention. And if I had said, "Wow! Just what I wanted. Thank you so much!" Luis would have felt momentarily gratified, but he would have understood that yes, he bought himself some time but only a facade of care.

The third decision point was telling Luis I loved him in our last session. It actually was not a risk, not because it was our last session but because the foundation of a trusting relationship with firm but not rigid boundaries had already been established. Luis would have known that I was lying if I had said that I cared about him only as I cared about all my patients, if I had said that caring was an important part of the therapy, or if I had said nothing at all. It would have been disingenuous, and I was not going to end our therapy that way. The regret is that we could have processed this together if I had brought it up earlier in the termination phase of therapy.

SUMMARY

This chapter focused on some of the potential pitfalls that can occur when sex is a topic in psychotherapy. The main concern and the most egregious form of harm are the sexual boundary violations that too often occur in therapy. When discussing sex in psychotherapy, it is imperative to ensure that the therapy is focused on the patient's needs and is in tune with what the patient has the ability to process in the moment. Avoiding the topic of sex does not guarantee that boundary violations will not occur. Sexual feelings and desires left unchecked can, in fact, lead to the slippery slope of violation and malpractice. Instead, to minimize the risk of harm and improve therapy outcomes, therapists can become more comfortable and adept at processing sexual content in psychotherapy. This would require understanding when and how to explore a patient's attraction, how to manage one's own attraction to a patient, how to handle the judicious use of self-disclosures, and when and how to ask about sexual fantasies.

PART II CLINICAL APPLICATIONS

4 SHAME

Doug was born with a misshapen penis. The shame of it bent and distorted the man he would become. At 15, Diane snuck out of the house to attend a party and was raped. The shame of it nearly killed her. Melanie discovered that sexually explicit pictures of her were shared among her boyfriend's friend group. The shame of it walled her off from the world.

Doug, Diane, and Melanie had never talked about their shame, and yet being sexual and enjoying sex were virtually impossible for all three of them. Doug came to therapy for depression. Diane came to therapy for anxiety. Melanie came to therapy for help with career decisions. All three had previously been in therapy and had never raised the subject of sex. Doug knew there was nothing to be done about his penis. So why talk about it? Diane was too ashamed and did not want her therapist to think badly of her. Melanie believed that she had "gotten over it" as she excelled at school and her career.

Therapy is supposed to be a safe place for people to share personal and sensitive information about themselves. After all, patients' disclosures are the source material for psychotherapy, and patient honesty would then seem to be a necessary touchstone. Strict boundaries and rules of confidentiality

https://doi.org/10.1037/0000483-005
Talking About Sex in Psychotherapy: A Guide for Every Therapist, by K. S. K. Hall

are in place to ensure that patients may reveal themselves without fear of judgment or repercussions. But in reality, patients often keep vital information to themselves for fear that they will be judged, that there will be repercussions, or because they do not see the necessity for divulging shameful secrets. This chapter alerts therapists to the importance of alleviating sexual shame. Helping patients talk openly and honestly in therapy about sexual feelings and behaviors is a fundamental therapeutic task.

SHAME ON YOU! SEX AND LIES IN PSYCHOTHERAPY

Farber, Blanchard, and Love (2019) have conducted a number of studies on deception, secret-keeping, and dishonesty in psychotherapy and have summarized and synthesized their own and others' research into a rather illuminating book: *Secrets and Lies in Psychotherapy*. In reviewing the literature, they conclude that somewhere between 83% and 94% of patients lie to their therapists, and that sexual issues are the most commonly endorsed topics of deception. They follow up these remarkable statistics with this rather shocking observation: "Simply put, the anticipation of shame is likely the greatest single deterrent to truth telling in psychotherapy" (Farber et al., 2019, p. 88). In other words, shame about sex deters honesty in psychotherapy. And honesty is a foundation of the process.

Despite the importance of shame in their work on deception, Farber and his colleagues (2019) do not define the emotion. Perhaps this is because we have all felt it—in its milder form of embarrassment, or in its stronger iterations of mortification and humiliation. But just so we all know what it is we are talking about in this chapter, the following description is helpful:

> Shame—a feeling of inferiority, inadequacy, incompetence, helplessness; a sense of self as defective, flawed, leading to a pervasive sense of failure, unworthiness, and to an experience of being scorned, unloved, and forsaken. . . . Shame leads to a wish to hide, to keep the flawed sense of self secret, and to avoid any interpersonal context that might reveal one's inadequacy and lead to further rejection. (Elise, 2008, p. 77)

One can see from this description that shame is a deterrent not only to going to therapy in the first place but also to successful therapy, especially to the integration of sexual issues into an understanding of the patient as a whole person. Shame may result from the way one is, as in Doug's case, or from what has happened to a person, as with Diane and Melanie, or from what a person has done, as was the situation with Chris, a man who was facing the loss of his marriage and family after the discovery of his numerous affairs.

ACTIVE DECEPTION

Diane, who sneaked out to a party and was raped, felt an incredible amount of shame about the whole event. She blamed herself for sneaking out. It was the reason, she told herself, that she could not report the rape to the police, despite the fact that she had bruises and lacerations from the assault. She blamed herself for being stupid, as if that was the reason she was raped. She told herself that it was best to forget it. Though she worried about having contracted an infection or becoming pregnant, she would not seek medical care because of the obvious injury to her genitals. Diane became studious, withdrawn, and serious throughout high school and college. When Diane came to therapy, she was highly anxious. Her presenting complaint was anxiety about urinary incontinence. She was a first-grade teacher and had become worried about losing control of her bladder during class time. She was unable to take bathroom breaks, except at lunch and during planned activities when the children left the classroom (art, gym). The anxiety was getting so severe that Diane was considering a career change. Her boyfriend convinced her to go to therapy. Reluctantly, she did.

Many cases in this book involve patients not revealing key aspects of their sexual lives in therapy. To call these deceptions feels too severe and judgmental. Most, if not all, of the patients do not see the link between their sexuality and their current presenting complaint, whereas others are optimistic that their problems can be resolved without needing to talk about shameful sexual topics, and still others wait to be asked about sex. Diane fell into two of the three categories. She hoped that she would never need to talk about sex because she did not see the connection between her current distress and her past sexual trauma. But Diane was also actively deceptive. I asked about sex. She lied.

"Why are you coming to therapy now?" This is a pretty standard question in many initial therapy encounters. Diane said that she was coming to therapy because the problem was getting worse and because her boyfriend encouraged her. "Has anything changed in your life?" Again, another standard question—to which Diane lied. "No, nothing I can think of." Since I routinely ask about sex, I gave Diane more opportunities for deception.

ME: Does your worry about incontinence affect you sexually?

DIANE: No.

ME: Not with intercourse or orgasm?

DIANE: We don't have intercourse. We're waiting for marriage.

ME: And orgasm? Alone or with your boyfriend?

DIANE: No, no problems. Just really at school. That's when I worry the most.

I did not press Diane further, although this presentation did not seem genuine to me. Her demeanor was more anxious during this exchange than it was previously in the session. Her answers also did not make much sense. Although waiting to have intercourse is an option for many people, especially those of certain religious faiths, it is an option that many people with anxiety opt for as well. I made a mental note to explore anxiety about sex. It also did not seem realistic that Diane had no concerns about losing bladder control when she had an orgasm. She did not say that she always empties her bladder before sex; rather, she dismissed any concerns related to sex. Again, I made a mental note. I did not push Diane during this session and subsequent ones. Until Diane and I had a stronger therapeutic alliance, I did not want her to feel the need to lie more. It does not feel good to lie, let alone to lie to your therapist. And although it is not a positive experience to be lied to as a therapist, it is helpful to know that it happens in the vast majority of cases.

TIMING IS EVERYTHING

Pacing and timing are incredibly important in the process of psychotherapy. Many patients need to be encouraged to share personal information, as it is a new experience (especially regarding sexual topics). Other patients want to tell you everything in that first session and sometimes need to be slowed down. A huge "data dump" can later be overwhelming, and patients may not want to return to therapy after having "said too much." But when you, as the therapist, have the impression that the patient is not being forthright and honest, it is a tricky balance to know when to confront and when to table it for later. A general rule of thumb may be to wait when shame and anxiety appear to be at the root of the secrecy. Sexual secrets take time and trust to be revealed.

Diane and I made some headway with her fears of incontinence. She was able to see that her thoughts were worries rather than premonitions, she made good use of strategies that helped give her confidence in her ability to control her bladder, and she confided in a coworker who said she would fill in if Diane needed to leave her classroom on short notice. Still, her anxiety was high, and she felt recurrently depressed and hopeless despite her progress.

Returning again to some of the earlier material that one has made a mental note of is helpful when therapy appears to be at a stalemate. I inquired about whether there were any changes in her sex life and whether these changes might also be affecting her worries about urinary incontinence.

ME: Is there any change when you and Philippe have sex?

DIANE: Well, we don't have sex.

ME: I know you don't have intercourse. I meant sex more broadly as any sexual activity.

DIANE: Oh, well, ya, no. No change.

ME: By the way, was it always your intention to wait until marriage to have intercourse?

DIANE: (*long pause*) Philippe is the first man I've ever really been serious with. We did try to have intercourse once. But it really hurt. A lot. So, we decided that perhaps it was best to wait until we were married. You know. Then sex would be guilt free.

ME: Oh, I'm sorry to hear that sex was painful. Did you go to a gynecologist to see if there was anything physical causing the pain?

DIANE: I don't have a gynecologist. I've never been.

The door was now slightly open. Diane was offering more information about sex. I later learned that the painful attempt to have intercourse happened just a week before Diane's anxiety about urinary incontinence became more severe. I mused that perhaps there is a link, that the feeling that there is something wrong with her body "down there" may have triggered the anxiety. I also noted that the anxiety occurs only when she feels trapped in her classroom. Diane was silent during my musing and looked stricken. Diane canceled the next session.

When Diane did come back to therapy, we talked about the link between the painful attempt at intercourse and her anxiety. Diane was apologetic and embarrassed about not telling me sooner. I normalized this ("You didn't necessarily know there was a link; it was a difficult topic, and some things take time to be revealed"). She was relieved that I was not angry with her and then told me the story about her rape, except in the first telling of it, she told me it was an attempted rape and it hurt. She told me that she sneaked out of her house to go to a party. Her parents had not wanted her to go because there would be drinking. She went anyway. She met a boy she did not know.

He took her to an upstairs bedroom and tried to rape her. She kept her legs clenched so tightly that he could not penetrate her. He left, disgusted and angry. She never saw him again.

I did not know then that the boy had, in fact, forcibly penetrated Diane and that she had lacerations from the violence of the attack. She had never had intercourse before, had never used a tampon, and had never had a gynecologic exam. She was not aroused or lubricated or physically ready for penetration. Likely, Diane had small tears around her vaginal opening, which accounted for the bleeding and the pain she experienced days afterward. But I did know that stories evolve in psychotherapy. I did know, as we have all experienced, that talking about events leads to an exploration of events—their impacts, their causes, and their importance. I remained open to hearing more and to hearing different versions of the story as we revisited it in therapy.

Diane finally told me about the rape and her anxiety about being damaged. She told me that she had waited downstairs at the party to use the toilet, but when she could not wait much longer, she ventured upstairs to find a bathroom. When she came out of the en suite bathroom in the master bedroom, the boy was waiting for her and raped her. Since that time, she has always needed to know she could get to a bathroom if she needed one. This is why the classroom presented such a problem.

But Diane had another concern. Waiting until marriage meant that intercourse would be attempted again once she was married. With Philippe talking about getting engaged soon, Diane was panicked. She hoped that by addressing her urinary anxiety, she would be able to manage her anxiety about sex as well. She hoped that by talking about an attempted rape, she could salvage some of her self-esteem and at least portray to me that she was not stupid and had been able to protect herself. When she finally disclosed the whole story, we were able to address her shame and anxiety in therapy.

It has been over 5 years now. Philippe is gone. He said he could not deal with the fact that she did not trust him enough to tell him about the rape, but Diane also recognizes that she has a lot of healing to do and that asking Philippe to understand and to put his own needs aside was a big ask. Diane has had a gynecologic exam, and she is physically healthy. She is currently going to a pelvic floor physical therapist to help with the tension in her pelvic floor (encompassing her vaginal opening and her urethral opening). She continues in therapy with me, and we are working on trust—trusting herself enough to know when to trust others—and we are working on seeing sex as an enjoyable activity. Diane is doing some exploration on her own as she would like to experience orgasm (never having had an orgasm is another thing that Diane lied to Philippe and to me about).

SHAME, GUILT, AND RELIGIOUS CONVICTION

In the 1960s, a young researcher named Donald Mosher did his doctoral dissertation on the propensity to experience guilt as a dimension of personality. He identified three subtypes of guilt—sex guilt, hostility guilt, and morality–conscience guilt—and developed a questionnaire for their measurement. Several revisions later, the Revised Mosher Guilt Inventory is still in use today (Mosher, 1966, 2019).

Although shame and guilt are frequent, if unhealthy, bedfellows, they differ in important ways. *Guilt* is typically a feeling that occurs following or in anticipation of a transgression. Anticipation of guilt can inhibit behavior, while the experience of guilt following a perceived transgression can be determined by confessions of wrongdoing, attempts at atonement, or self-punishment (Abramson et al., 1977). Mosher was particularly interested in measuring the personality disposition toward guilt while recognizing that guilt can also be a transitory state of being, an emotional experience involving regret and remorse. *Shame*, on the other hand, is not linked to a transgression but is an emotional and negative evaluation of the self. Where guilt says, "I did a bad thing," shame says, "I am bad."

A disposition toward experiencing guilt is not universally considered a negative personality trait. Sexually conservative cultures and religions view a propensity to experience sex guilt as a positive quality, given that such guilt would likely prevent engaging in what are considered wrong sexual behaviors (e.g., premarital sex; Maarefi et al., 2020). Indeed, many religiously observant patients experience their guilt as a helpful guide for making important life and sexual choices.

Religiosity (strong religious beliefs and convictions) has been linked to poor sexual satisfaction because of its inhibiting effects on sexual behavior, sexual exploration, and sexual pleasure (Fortenberry & Hensel, 2022). Sex guilt is often cited as a mediating variable responsible for this effect (Emmers-Sommer et al., 2018). Given the importance of their faith, it is difficult to directly intervene to reduce sex guilt and increase sexual pleasure in highly religious patients through cognitive behavior interventions, including confronting cognitive distortions and prescribing pleasurable sexual activities. However, by highlighting the spiritual aspect of sex, it has been proposed that "religiosity could positively influence sexual satisfaction by imbuing the sexual relationship with a sanctified, divine sense of meaning" (Leonhardt et al., 2020, p. 214). While there is currently no evidence that this approach is effective, it does offer an intriguing clinical pathway. It makes intuitive sense that helping religiously observant patients experience sexual joy and pleasure from the sexual activities that are sanctioned by their faith will yield better results than trying to loosen their reliance on their faith to guide their sexual choices.

When guilt is internalized and generalized to become an overall negative appraisal of the self, it marks the beginnings of shame. Guilt is an emotional experience, a temporary state resulting from a transgression, whereas shame is enduring and omnipresent.

THE OMNIPRESENT EMBODIMENT OF SHAME

Diane was ashamed that she had been raped. When she first encountered the boy in the bedroom, she was pleased to think he had followed her upstairs, finding her attractive. She enjoyed making out with him on the bed. But when it turned ugly and violent, the shame of being vulnerable, of being initially pleased and aroused, was internalized in her psyche and in her body. And she wanted to hide from the shame, so she did not tell anyone and she avoided sex and sexual pleasure. Every time Diane started to feel sexual pleasure in her body, she would also have a sick feeling—a feeling of shame—so, to avoid the feeling, she avoided sex.

Melanie discovered that the boyfriend she trusted had shared sexually explicit photographs of her. She imagined the mocking laughter of her boyfriend and his friends and assumed they critiqued every inch of her exposed body. Her humiliation consumed her, and instead of experiencing attraction and arousal when she encountered interested men, she felt a burning pit in her gut. She felt shame throughout her body. As a result, Melanie avoided interacting with men in social situations and instead limited herself to church and work, places where her spirituality and intellect would be prized over her now-neglected body (Melanie neither exercised nor ate a healthy diet). In fact, Melanie mostly felt nothing in her numbed and steeled body. So, when faced with a big career decision involving a move overseas, she did not know how to make the choice. To go or not to go? How did she feel about it? She did not know, and countless pros and cons lists were not helping. Her avoidance of her embodied shame had generalized to the extent that she felt nothing at all. She could not access her feelings when she needed to make a choice based on what she wanted rather than what was right.

SHAME IS IN OUR SKILL SET

Exploring sexual topics, especially shameful sexual topics, requires the skills and sensitivities that therapists have training in. We are taught to listen to our patients' stories, and we develop a way of experiencing and understanding our patients while maintaining a perspective that often differs from theirs. For example, we understand and empathize when our patients are hopeless. But we do not agree with them that they are hopeless or that their lives or situations are hopeless. When people present with sexual distress, they often feel hopeless, as they have tried on their own, but without success, to resolve their problems. Sometimes we empathize with our patients' embarrassment regarding their sexual thoughts, feelings, and behaviors (past and present), but we do not need to agree that their sexuality is inherently embarrassing or shameful. Our helping instincts often tempt us to alleviate shame quickly, but shame will not be so easily disposed of. Shame festers in secrecy, and the very bold act of bringing shame into the open in psychotherapy is tremendously healing.

Douglas felt hopeless because he was born with a condition known as hypospadias, in which the opening of the urethra is on the underside of the penis, and the penis is often curved (as it was in Douglas's case). Surgery to correct the defect in infancy was not successful for Douglas, and he spent his life feeling inadequate as a man. His shame made him needy and angry, and while he longed for a relationship with a woman, he inevitably devalued any woman interested in him. He came to therapy on the brink of divorce from his second wife. Unlike Diane and Melanie, Douglas told me immediately about the source of his shame—his hypospadias—and then he was openly hostile when I told him I did not know what it was.

DOUGLAS: You're a specialist in sex, and you don't know this?

ME: No, tell me about it.

DOUGLAS: Look (*drawing a picture of a crooked penis*), that's what my dick looks like. I can't pee standing up. I can't fuck like a normal guy. It's bent, and my urethra's on the side, not the top.

ME: It's important to you that I know this about you upfront. (I am consciously ignoring his apparent anger and disdain. I believe it is a defense against his shame, and we will work on this later in therapy.)

DOUGLAS: I just want to get it out of the way.

ME: Tell me how it has affected your life, your marriage.

DOUGLAS: She knew about it before, so it isn't the problem. She says the problem is my attitude and the way I treat people. Her family mainly. But they're a bunch of assholes, and I can't tolerate assholes.

Douglas's wife did divorce him. He was indeed horribly abusive to her family and friends, and to her. Anytime he felt shame, he countered with aggression. Initially, he resisted any attempts I made to connect his hostility to his shame. However, over the course of many years of therapy, Douglas slowly began to open up about how badly he felt about himself, how humiliated he felt because he could not use a urinal, how he was bullied by his male classmates, and how vulnerable he had to be during sex, as intercourse required careful positioning. Over the years, especially after his wife left him, he felt hopeless and suicidal. He was hopeless about the possibility of being loved, and of course, the way he behaved made that possibility even more remote.

Throughout, I empathized with his sense of powerlessness and his sense of shame, but I did not agree with him that his bent penis made him less of a man. I did not condone his behavior when he picked fights with strangers, ogled women, and generally behaved poorly, even though I understood the pain beneath it. As therapy progressed, I could see that Douglas's shame was subsiding. He was kinder and more aware of the feelings and sensibilities of others. He began to date again. Sadly, Douglas was diagnosed with pancreatic cancer and died a few months after his diagnosis. In the last few months of his life, he was full of regret and remorse for how he had behaved during his lifetime. Our last meeting took place 3 days before he died. He was in hospice care. His nurses thought he was a wonderful man. He thanked me for "trying to help me get it right."

Douglas was a patient for life, someone who would likely always need the support and insights of a caring, trusted therapist to better navigate a life built on shame. Long-term therapy patients are often a challenge, as progress can be slow, and gains may be reversed at times. Douglas's life was shortened by his cancer, and he recognized in death that he had not yet "got it right," but he had come a long way in order to treat his female nurses with gratitude and to also recognize and thank me for my efforts.

KEEPING THE SHAME

In Chapter 2, we discussed referring patients for specialized treatment. But as these cases demonstrate, there is potential for harm when referring out. Diane required the trust built through long-term therapy to open up about her assault and then to help her navigate the medical care and attention she needed. Switching therapists would have been detrimental to her sense of self, her ability to trust, and her progress, to say the least. Once Melanie began to open up to her feelings, her feelings of shame flooded her. Melanie turned down the opportunity to work overseas, knowing that she had work to do in therapy and did not want to start over with a new therapist.

Douglas was full of shame, and his defensiveness often made it difficult to be in the room with him. I was unfamiliar with hypospadias when I first encountered Douglas. I learned most about his experience with hypospadias by being open about my ignorance and asking him to tell me about his condition. I also consulted medical texts. Referring Douglas to a specialist (if there were such a person) would have furthered his sense of shame and his belief that his misshapen penis was at the root of all rejections. In fact, educating ourselves about our patients' medical/sexual conditions may enhance treatment progress. For example, I told Douglas, "I have been reading about hypospadias, and I read that fertility is sometimes an issue. Is that true for you?" Douglas was gratified that I had taken the interest to do research on his condition. From a position of naivete and curiosity, I could also introduce questions that furthered our work in therapy, for example, examining other aspects of masculinity (virility, potential fatherhood).

SHAME ON ME

Shame, of course, is not limited to our patients. As therapists, we may carry our own sense of shame, perhaps in its milder iteration of embarrassment. We may be embarrassed not to have expertise or expert knowledge, especially about sexuality. In fact, of the reasons patients do not talk about sex, one is the fear that the therapist will be judgmental and shaming, but another is the belief that the therapist will be ineffective, will avoid the topic, or will be uncomfortable (Farber et al., 2019). So, while some patients doubt that their therapist can help them or understand their sexual concerns, other patients attribute their inhibition to therapist technique—describing their therapists as either failing to understand and empathize or engaging in marked avoidance of sexual topics. Patients may shy away not only from topics that are embarrassing to them but also from topics that might be embarrassing to us, their therapists. Farber and his colleagues noted that, in retrospect, none of the participants in their studies felt that dishonesty or avoidance of sexual topics was helpful to their progress.

Our shame about sex may extend beyond the embarrassment of not knowing enough. As with the patients I have discussed in this chapter, we may embody the shame of sexual things we have done, of sexual things done to us, or of who we are as sexual beings (e.g., we may feel unattractive sexually or feel ashamed of our kinky sexual preferences, our choice of partner, or our sexual inadequacy). Shame works on therapists the same way it does for everyone else. It is an embodied emotional experience that makes us want to hide. Even if we are well aware of the source of our shame, we may yet be wholly or partially unaware of how it affects our clinical work.

As you reflect on your work with patients, past and present, you may notice the feeling of shame (whether a burning in your gut, a pit in your stomach, or the uncomfortable warmth of a blush spreading across your skin) when sex is a topic in therapy. Please consider that your shame is likely being perceived by your patients as being about them. Also consider that you cannot deeply explore your patients' sexual shame if you are mired in yours. As you work through your issues in your own therapy and supervision, tolerating and attending to the shame you presently experience in the moment in psychotherapy is necessary. I have sometimes taken deep breaths and have occasionally given myself a surreptitious pinch if I feel shame mounting. And then I consciously and deliberately refocus on my patient.

THE GIFT OF UNDERSTANDING

As therapists, we must understand that most patients withhold information or outright lie in therapy, and much of the withheld information pertains to sex. The opportunity to talk about the source of their shame with a helpful, compassionate, and knowledgeable therapist is a gift, because the unburdening replaces shame with compassion and understanding, talking honestly is a relief, and the process of sharing greatly enhances the progress of treatment. Farber et al. (2019) note that deception occurs "without great forethought and, to a great degree, early on in the therapeutic relationship" (p. 134). Thus, circling back to topics, especially those related to sex, and providing opportunities to reconsider or amend disclosures can be important techniques to add to therapy.

In his wonderful book *The Gift of Therapy*, Irvin Yalom (2002) offers another pathway to explore hidden secrets in psychotherapy. He states that there "is always some concealment, some information withheld because of shame, because of some particular way they wish me to regard them" (Yalom, 2002, p. 74). So, when his patients describe an act of concealment outside of therapy, he invites an exploration of concealment within the therapeutic relationship as well.

Chris came to see me after what he called "D-Day," or the day his wife discovered his numerous extramarital affairs, as well as money spent on sex workers and pornography subscriptions. Chris came to see me when he had fallen far from the heights he had imagined for himself. Rich, successful, and "happily" married, he was on top of the world, and then he was not. I knew that Chris would not want to enter therapy as an abject failure. I knew that he would want me to regard him well but worry that I would judge him and perhaps not even help him. So, I knew that he would want to present himself in a favorable light and that there was a strong likelihood that there would be errors of omission when telling me his story. I did not challenge him on this early on in therapy, not before we had a strong therapeutic alliance. Here is an interaction that occurred several months into our therapy together:

CHRIS: I'll never earn my wife's trust back. Never. She thinks I'm a liar. I guess I am. She thinks once a liar, always a liar.

ME: What do you think—once a liar and all that—what do you think?

CHRIS: I don't know. I lied for so long. She's not wrong, you know. I lied. A lot.

ME: I think that people lie for many reasons. Sometimes they believe—rightly or wrongly—that they are protecting the ones they love. Sometimes they lie to make a good impression, and sometimes people get caught in lies—and then have to keep lying. (*Chris nods and looks down rather glumly at his feet.*) It's likely that's happened here between you and me, that there have been some things that have been hard for you to be completely truthful about, and if it hasn't happened, it could.

CHRIS: No, no. I've always been completely honest with you. I mean, this is therapy. You're supposed to be completely honest, right? What would be the point of lying to you?

ME: I just want us to be aware that there may come a point in time when it will be hard to be honest, even in therapy. We are doing good work together, and you may be fearful of jeopardizing that or you may worry that you will disappoint me.

CHRIS: Oh, don't worry. I've always been completely honest with you, and I know that's the deal. I'm not going to lie in therapy.

I did not point out to Chris that honesty was "the deal" in his marriage as well. But despite his protests, my words sank in. Over the next several sessions, he "spontaneously" amended some of his earlier stories, saying he forgot, he just remembered, or to clarify . . . Chris was working hard in therapy. It was a risk for him, to bring himself fully to a relationship. Almost a year later, Chris told me that he had gone to a sex worker again. He said he contemplated not telling me, but then he said that he remembered our conversation about honesty in therapy. As he found himself justifying the choice to lie to me (she'll be disappointed, it's just one time, and I won't do it again), he knew he had said these words before when he was justifying lying to his wife. Chris's honesty allowed us to more fully understand his dynamics: that when he feared losing a valuable connection, he turned to sex to relieve his anxiety and to feel attached to someone, at least for one brief moment. Therapy allowed Chris to forge a connection with a stable other person, to experiment with truth, and ultimately to be truthful, which gave him a solid base to navigate future relationships, including a reconciliation with his wife, which he had not thought possible.

SHAME AND SEXUAL FANTASIES

Often the manifestation of shame occurs in secret sexual fantasies. While there is evidence that sexual shame as a result of experiencing nonconsensual sexual experiences (including childhood sexual abuse, incest, sexual harassment, assault, and rape) affects sexual experiences in adulthood (Pulverman & Meston, 2020), little is known about how shame affects sexual fantasies. Sexual fantasies are extremely difficult for people to discuss. Decades ago, Nancy Friday (1973, 1980) wrote groundbreaking books in which she compiled the sexual fantasies of men and women. While not scientific, the books served notice that sexual fantasies do not necessarily reflect sexual wishes and demonstrated a broad range of fantasies from the mundane to the taboo.

In my own clinical experience, patients are reluctant to reveal their sexual fantasies unless the fantasies are distressing to them. Still, they worry that these fantasies, the very ones that are distressing but at the same time compellingly arousing, will signal to the therapist that there is something very wrong with them. Women and men who have been sexually abused have reported having intrusive thoughts of their abuse during consensual sexual activities. They also describe masturbating to abuse fantasies as well (Gewirtz-Meydan & Opuda, 2023). But without a trauma history, some patients are perplexed as to why they are fantasizing about activities that they would never want to engage in, or indeed that they find repugnant. The shameful answer many come up with is something like "I must be sick, perverted. I must secretly really want these things."

Marc was raised by his paternal grandmother after his heroin-addicted father died of AIDS and after his mother essentially abandoned him to have a new life in California. He lived with his mother for several months after his father's funeral; then she left him, at the age of 12, with his grandmother because she was "going on a trip." Thereafter, he received an occasional birthday card and finally a phone call from her when he turned 21. He has a tepid relationship with his mother now. But Marc, currently in his early 40s, has never dated, has never had sex with anyone, and is committed to a life alone. He had been in therapy previously, working on "my abandonment issues." But what brought him to therapy now was his concern about his sexual fantasies. In his fantasies, he is forced to dress in women's clothing, then he must serve an anonymous group of men (performing menial tasks for them), and finally he is forced to submit sexually to one of the men. He finds these fantasies disgusting, repugnant, vile, and sexually exciting. From adolescence onward, these fantasies have accompanied him when he masturbated. He is repulsed and aroused by these fantasies, and he is sure that they make him unfit to have a relationship. Now in his early 40s, he wants to make one last-ditch effort.

It was extraordinarily painful for Marc to share these fantasies in therapy. And make no mistake, they were difficult to hear. In graphic detail, Marc described both his sexual fantasies and the utter humiliation and shame he felt in the fantasies, as well as the shame he experienced after he ejaculated. These disclosures occurred over many sessions. Marc felt the shame as he was in the sessions with me. It was painful. Therapy was a slow process as we tried to understand the fantasies almost as we would have tried to decipher the meaning of a distressing dream. This effort helped Marc see the fantasies as something other than an indication of his extreme depravity. He had already tried, without success, to alter his fantasies or to stop fantasizing altogether, and he even tried to stop masturbating. He felt hopeless. Sharing his fantasies in therapy was a first for Marc, and having a compassionate listener was a new experience for him.

We came to understand that Marc channeled his sense of shame into his sexual fantasies in an attempt to express his forbidden feelings. Marc was ashamed that his father was a drug addict, he was ashamed that his father was HIV positive, and when his father developed AIDS and was hospitalized, Marc was discouraged from seeing him by his mother and grandmother. Letters to him from his father as he was dying went unanswered. Marc's shame about abandoning his father was compounded by his mother's abandonment of him and the extreme disapproval of his grandmother toward both his parents. He felt that he was not allowed to love or grieve for the loss of either his father or his mother. Instead, the shame that he was unlovable (his mother left him) and the shame he felt for abandoning his father made him feel undeserving of love and pleasure in life. Therefore, he could experience orgasm only when he was servile and humiliated, and because of these fantasies, he had the shame of being a sexual pervert.

It is important to note that not everyone who has humiliation fantasies has psychopathology or experiences shame. In Marc's case, there was a link, but this will not be true in every instance. It is a mistake to assume pathology based on a fantasy. We do not know enough about what makes a fantasy erotic to someone, but there are many people who enjoy fantasies of servitude and who are not suffering from any concomitant psychopathology.

Telling me his fantasies without being pathologized or rejected helped Marc. Having other ways of viewing his fantasies (expression of shame vs. an indication of perversion) also alleviated some of his shame-based depression. In eroticizing his shame, Marc was attempting to gain mastery over it.

Marc did start to date women but was unable to be sexual with any of them. He denied sexual attraction to men. To be truthful, I am not sure about Marc's sexual orientation (gay, straight, bisexual). If and when Marc explores relationships, his sexual orientation may become clearer. At present, Marc is focused instead on making life decisions that bring him pleasure rather than always trying to do the right thing to make up for how badly he feels. He has embarked on a career change and is trying to develop a group of friends.

Marc had been in therapy with a number of other therapists and had never managed to talk about his fantasies. This time in therapy, he knew he had to start by disclosing his fantasies before he began to care too much about what the therapist would think of him. Many patients will do what Marc did previously. They will start therapy with the hope of being able to reveal their fantasies, and they will likely make some effort to do so. It will take a skillful and astute therapist to pick up on the timid gestures. And on the rare occasions when the gestures are bolder, it takes a courageous therapist to follow up. Jumping in quickly to reassure ("It's normal to have taboo sexual fantasies") is, in fact, a way of cutting off therapeutic exploration of the sexual material. As we will learn throughout this book, listening to our patients' sexual stories is challenging but will ultimately lead to a fuller understanding of the person or couple in front of you. This, in turn, is likely to enhance the therapy outcome.

Our patients' distress about violent fantasies and their strong intention never to engage in the violence may comfort therapists who worry that their patients will harm others. When I worked with serial rapists, it was their lack of distress regarding their fantasies and behaviors and their lack of appreciation for another's feelings that were problematic. Here we are talking about patients who are reluctant to disclose fantasies because of their distress about harming others and their acute awareness of how they might be perceived by another person (the therapist). In fact, helping patients not to feel ashamed of themselves and to help them connect empathically and intimately with others will do more to prevent acting out than shaming them about their thoughts (Cantor, 2014; Ward, 2002).

BECOMING SHAMELESS

Shame—from childhood to one's last days—is a first-rate form of social control. Shame is what keeps us in line, and what prevents us from discovering not so much who we are, but what we might become.

—Bronski, 2004, p. xvi

Michael Bronski (2004) wrote these lines in his foreword to Patrick Moore's book *Beyond Shame: Reclaiming the Abandoned History of Radical Gay Sexuality*, which, among other things, presents the provocative idea that for the gay community to fight shame (shame about sex, shame about AIDS), a return to sex "as liberation and as joy" (p. xx) is necessary. The idea that sex can counter shame when shame is a primary tool for controlling sexuality is both exciting and intriguing. It is the basis of gay pride parades, drag queen story hours, and other acts of shamelessness. Many of the derogatory terms applied to people who engage in transgressive sex—from *slut* to *fag*, *pervert*, and more—have been reclaimed and repurposed by the people they were meant to shame as labels of pride instead.

Shaming as an attempt to control is often driven by fear. "Yes, okay. I understand that you are gay, but do you have to put it in everyone's face? Shouldn't sex be private?" People who are heterosexual can believe that sexuality should be private, because heterosexuality, considered the normative orientation in all parts of the world, is not a private sexual orientation at all. It is reflected in many layers of our culture (think about media representations of couples; think about government laws that privilege heterosexual couples; reflect on the fairy tales and children's stories you read; and remember your sex education classes and, if you participated, your religious education). Shame makes you want to hide, and shame festers in private. So pride parades, kink festivals, and other ways of putting nonnormative sexuality "in our faces" are acts of personal, political, and psychological rebellion. They are repudiations of shame.

We can accomplish something similar in our work with sexual minority patients by bringing the topic of sex out into the open and safe space of psychotherapy. Many will come to psychotherapy with shame about their sexuality. Many will have been shamed for their sexual orientation, their sexual expressions, and their sexual behavior. Actively encouraging our patients to talk about sex, especially their sexual secrets, bestows the gift of acceptance and understanding. There are several ways in which this is accomplished. One is very subtle but foundational: an attitude of openness and acceptance. Other ways involve the questions we ask, how we ask them, and how we respond. You will read many examples in this book, and you can look back at the examples in Chapter 2, but a general rule is to be inquisitive and nonjudgmental. Remember that you do not need to be a sex expert. You are not required to render an opinion on normalcy or healthiness. You need to be open and curious and help the patient more fully understand their sexuality so they can make their own sexual decisions.

SHAME AND UNCERTAINTY IN SEXUAL MINORITIES

People are shamed for deviating from the norm. It follows then that the farther the deviation, the greater the shaming. Sexual minorities will experience more traumatic shaming experiences than will heteronormative individuals and couples. These shaming experiences will negatively affect their mental health, while encountering compassionate and supportive people and actions will mitigate these effects (Seabra et al., 2023). Understanding the challenges of sexual minority patients in context is key. Any change in more overtly expressing their sexuality may risk the loss of important relationships (with parents, partners, friends, and institutions such as churches, schools, and occupational settings) that are holding them together psychologically. Proceed, but proceed with care and caution.

Wyatt came to see me in his late twenties in a state of confusion. He believed that he had finally come to accept a female gender identity that he had previously felt too ashamed to acknowledge. He had also recently started a heterosexual relationship with a cisgender woman whom he really cared about. It was his first romantic relationship and his first sexual experience with a partner. When he confided his gender uncertainty to his girlfriend, she encouraged him to seek therapy because she loved him as a man.

After a few sessions with Wyatt, I was confused about the path forward, so I sought consultation with a psychotherapist with years of experience working with trans youth and adults. She was alarmed that Wyatt was beginning his transitional journey late in life and advised me that I should encourage him to begin the process, as his transition would be more difficult the longer he waited. In my next session with Wyatt, I gave him information about groups for transgender individuals that were meeting in the area. I also gave him the contact information for physicians who could prescribe hormones if he was ready for that step. I thought I was being gentle and helpful. After all, I was simply providing information. But in retrospect, I was advocating for Wyatt to change. I was confused about Wyatt's clinical presentation, and uncomfortable in my confusion, I sought consultation. But I sought consultation from an advocate for trans rights, and ultimately, I traded her certainty for my confusion. After that "gentle information" session, Wyatt never returned to therapy with me. I am deeply sad about that. I was influenced by the advocacy happening in my professional community and by the advocacy of the clinician consultant. I opted for certainty instead of understanding that my confusion was also Wyatt's confusion. I needed to tolerate the shame of feeling inadequate (to help Wyatt) and actually stay present to help Wyatt find his own path forward in his own time frame.

Looking back, I wonder whether Wyatt fully understood his feelings about his gender and sexuality, but I do know that he needed to work through the possibility of losing his one and only girlfriend if and when he transitioned. I hope that Wyatt found a path forward, hopefully with the help of a more patient therapist. But my mistake with Wyatt has helped me slow down and tolerate confusion and uncertainty in therapy. I am a better therapist because of it. But I do regret that I was not a better therapist for Wyatt.

SUMMARY

Sexual shame is perhaps the single greatest deterrent to the effective process and outcome of psychotherapy. We need to be aware that our patients will, more often than not, give us incomplete or inaccurate pictures of themselves as they begin therapy, and that these inaccuracies or omissions will likely relate to the experience of shame regarding sex. It takes time and trust for patients to fully and honestly reveal themselves in therapy. We must be aware that patients will lie or omit important information, usually about sex. We can provide opportunities for patients to revisit and repair and reflect upon any deceptions, omissions, and evasions that occurred earlier in the course of therapy. Shame is in our skill set. Bringing shame out into the open in the safe space of therapy is tremendously healing. We can empathize with our patients' experiences of shame without agreeing that they should be ashamed. We can help our patients see themselves in a different light. Working with shame takes time and patience. The rush to certainty, reassurance, or a quick fix is as countertherapeutic as silence.

5 DILEMMAS OF DESIRE

Desire is a longing for someone or something. Desire implies distance in time or space (or both) between us and who or what we desire. *Wanting*, *longing*, and *yearning* are words for poets but are often aversive states for people. We are impatient when we have to wait in line, we are testy when our computers take more than a second or two to download a file, and we search for online shopping sites that offer free overnight or even same-day delivery. We buy on credit because we do not want to wait. But with intimate partnered sex, sometimes, often, usually, we have to wait—we may need to wait to find a partner, we may need to wait for our partner to be interested in having sex, and we may need to wait until we both have time to have sex. This waiting period can be filled with pleasurable anticipation, anxiety-ridden dread, or despair that sex is never going to happen.

Whether and how sexual desire is experienced and expressed reflects how our patients relate to themselves and others. Do they feel desirable (worthwhile, attractive, loveable)? How do they respond to their partner's desire (dread, desire, duty)? Do they feel entitled to want, to desire? And what happens when one must wait or do without?

In this chapter, the mirror of sexuality is more than a metaphor. It is an important therapeutic tool. Our patients' relationship with their sexuality

https://doi.org/10.1037/0000483-006
Talking About Sex in Psychotherapy: A Guide for Every Therapist, by K. S. K. Hall

and how that sexuality is expressed can provide an important avenue for insight into our patients' psyches. More than a simple reflection, however, the mirror of sexuality often magnifies psychological dynamics that might otherwise be difficult to discern. Our patients' sexuality can provide a pathway for treatment, opening up options that would otherwise not be available for addressing our patients' presenting problems. Addressing sexual issues can, for example, enhance communication, trust, and self-esteem, which are the bedrocks for many other issues that our patients face.

In this chapter, I discuss two cases that present views from both sides of the mirror that sexuality offers. In the first case, Selby came to therapy for help dealing with the stresses in her life. How she managed those stresses provided insight into her difficulties with sexual desire when she embarked on a new relationship several months into her therapy. In the second case, we are looking from the other side of the mirror, from sexuality to other life difficulties. Grant came to therapy with a presenting complaint of low sexual desire, and it was the insight provided by his almost-absent desire for partnered sex that revealed the difficulties that Grant covered up in the rest of his life.

MANAGING LOW DESIRE

Selby's life was complicated. She wanted a career as a photographer but years ago took a well-paying job in a marketing agency where she was eventually promoted to management. Selby hated managing others. She had a mother who was addicted to prescription pain medication, a father who was an enabler, a sister who was disengaged, a brother who was incarcerated, and a boyfriend (Ethan) who was unhappy. So, although Selby "hated" it, in most of her significant relationships, she found herself in the position of "manager."

Selby came to therapy with low self-esteem, chronic dysphoria, and episodic anxiety. A single woman in her early 30s, she had a careworn expression and large, watchful eyes. She was attractive, but you could tell by the way she carried herself that she did not take pride in her appearance. Several months into her therapy, Selby was excited to be dating Ethan and was hopeful this relationship would work out. However, several months after meeting him, it was Ethan's unhappiness about their sex life that took center stage in Selby's therapy: "I don't want to lose him," Selby said.

I quickly discovered that Selby's approach to her relationship with her boyfriend, overall and sexually, was to manage. I quickly recognized this pattern, as it had been a focus of our work regarding her family issues. I was not surprised that Selby interpreted her role as being the one to "fix"

Ethan. Ethan, as viewed through Selby's eyes (how else would I come to know him?), was in need. Recently divorced due to his wife's infidelity, poor Ethan needed a self-esteem boost. He needed the reassurance of Selby's desire, pleasure, and orgasm. And Selby was wondering why she could not provide this for Ethan. What was wrong with her that she could not find sexual desire for a man she loves? Although Selby was distressed by her lack of desire for Ethan, she recognized her pattern of losing desire in intimate relationships: "Maybe I'm asexual?" she wondered.

The Umbrella of Asexuality

Asexuality is a matter of self-identification that has some individuals, like Selby, questioning whether the label might fit them. Essentially, *asexuality* is a sexual orientation and an umbrella designation for absent, low, or variable sexual attraction to others. While most people think of asexuals as having no interest in sex whatsoever, under the umbrella of asexuality are various subgroups such as demisexuals, who require a strong emotional bond before experiencing any attraction, and gray asexuals, or gray As, who may experience attraction very infrequently (e.g., several times a year) or weakly, or only under very specific circumstances (Nimbi et al., 2024).

Selby did her own research and thought that perhaps she was a gray asexual—or, more specifically, a member of a subgroup of the grays—a fraysexual—someone whose sexual attraction fades once they get to know someone. Selby reported that her sexual interest in Ethan diminished as the relationship became more intimate, in other words, as she got to know him better. But was Selby attracted only to strangers, or as I wondered, did this pattern of losing interest reveal underlying anxiety with increasing relational intimacy?

Adding to the complexity of the issue for Selby is the fact that asexuals (or Aces, as they are colloquially known) may engage in sex (recall from Chapter 1 that sexual attraction and desire are not the only motivations for sexual activity). So, the fact that Selby had sex with Ethan on a regular, if infrequent (according to Ethan), basis did not rule out asexuality. Asexuals can and often do experience arousal and orgasm during sex, and asexual individuals also masturbate. Asexuality is a sexual orientation that indicates a lack of sexual attraction to others, not a deficit in physiological sexual responding (Brotto & Yule, 2017).

Needing a physical release is the reason many asexuals give for engaging in solo sex, which is often done in a perfunctory manner without fantasy (Hermann et al., 2020; Hille et al., 2020). Here, too, Selby differed from asexuals. Selby rarely felt aroused and did not experience orgasm during partnered sex. Often, she felt discomfort and mild pain when she and Ethan were having intercourse, indicating that Selby was not even getting physically aroused during sex with Ethan. And Selby rarely, if ever, masturbated, despite the fact that she was reliably orgasmic when she did. Selby felt she needed to save whatever sexual energy she had for Ethan.

Selby genuinely wondered whether she was asexual, but she also hoped that being asexual would provide her some defense against Ethan's relentless criticisms regarding her lack of sexual interest in him. He would often complain that she was "cold" or "frigid," and he nicknamed her "Frosted Flakes." If she was asexual, Selby could say, "It's not my fault." I encouraged Selby not to apply labels too quickly but to tolerate uncertainty and ambiguity as we explored her sexuality/asexuality. I also observed that the nickname seemed unkind, but Selby shrugged it off.

The Wrong Question

"What is wrong with you?" was Ethan's frequent criticism, and Selby questioned as well, "What is wrong with me that I don't desire a man I love?" This is, of course, the wrong question. It leads Selby down a familiar path where the resounding answer is invariably "You're not good enough." (After all, isn't her inadequacy at the root of why she cannot fix her family?) A more helpful question for Selby to consider was "What is my lack of desire for Ethan telling me?" This is a sleight of hand, if you will, that therapists do all the time. We want to help our patients ask more meaningful questions, rather than continue to denigrate themselves with negative self-statements disguised as questions. But it was hard to get Selby to switch gears.

What did Selby talk about in therapy? She talked about many things: her unhappiness at work, her concern for her mother, and her despair that no one was stepping in to intervene. But when Selby talked about her relationship with Ethan, she talked about feeling guilty. Selby felt that it was her fault that Ethan was unhappy: "Of course he is unhappy! He's not getting sex!" I gently mentioned to Selby that she seemed to be feeling overly responsible, and I asked what Ethan was doing to try to improve their sexual relationship. In answer, I got a blank stare: "He can't do anything because I don't want to have sex!" To be fair, many low-desiring partners attribute their partners' unhappiness to the lack of sex: "Of course he yells at me—he's not getting sex!" Sadly, some low-desiring partners apply the same rationale to their partner's more extreme abusive behavior.

Selby had sex with Ethan because it had been a long time, because she knew him well enough to know that 10 days is about the maximum length of time he could go without having sex before becoming angry, sullen, and withdrawn. So she tried to get ahead of the game, and by Day 8 or 9, she was initiating sex. But her sexual initiation was disconnected from her sexual desires. She was not looking for times when she might feel a flicker of interest, or when she might feel close and want more intimacy with Ethan. Selby was scanning for his irritation and unhappiness, and when she found evidence of it, she initiated sex she did not want to have. Consequently, having the sex she did not want to have, Selby hurried through it. "Never mind me," she told Ethan. "There's no point trying to arouse me. Let's just focus on you." So Selby hurried through the sex she did not want to have by stimulating Ethan to arousal and erection, and with the help of a lubricant, they would have intercourse. Ethan would ejaculate. Mission accomplished; crisis averted. Except there was nothing in that scenario that would have the remotest chance of allowing Selby to enjoy her sexual experience with Ethan, so that perhaps once the sex started, it would be pleasurable, and maybe desire would even kick in to provide a whisper: "More, different, better, please." Recall the Basson model (Basson, 2001) from Chapter 1. Desire is not just a phase that precedes sexual activity. It is better understood as a companion throughout sex, guiding and motivating what you want next and building on the pleasure you are experiencing now.

The way that Selby approached sex is not unusual for people with little or no desire for the sex they are having. They time sex to avert their partner's unhappiness rather than paying attention to what might possibly put them in the mood (e.g., time spent talking or laughing together or a special occasion). And they rush through sex hoping to get it over with quickly, so they do not pay attention to any inkling of desire for sexual stimulation themselves. When this scenario is repeated too often—in other words, when people repeatedly consent to having sex they do not want—they can develop an aversion to sex. An aversion to sex is a visceral response of disgust that can finally render sex without desire a truly negative experience.

Her Hormones: It's Complicated

Selby thought she knew the message her body was sending her ("There is something psychologically wrong with you"), so she was not concerned about whether hormones were to blame for her low sexual desire. She was too young for menopause, and she had experienced low desire since her teenage years. She had been on and off various oral contraceptives over the years, and although she heard they could contribute to low desire, for Selby the protection from pregnancy more than made up for any hormonal problems (Caruso et al., 2022). And while some research shows that sexual desire can peak for women around ovulation (Marcinkowska et al., 2023),

Selby had never noticed any impact of her menstrual cycle on her desire or lack of desire for sex.

Hormones have a complicated relationship with female sexual desire. Oral contraceptives, menstrual cycle irregularities, and menopause (naturally occurring or surgically induced by the removal of the ovaries) may all trigger concern about a hormonal imbalance (and a consult with a gynecologist or sexual medicine specialist may be in order). If we refer back to the dual control model introduced in the first chapter, which described excitatory and inhibitory factors contributing to or detracting from desire and arousal, we can understand that a reduction in physiologically mediated levels of sexual desire (excitatory factors) will allow for anxiety (and other psychological inhibitors) to take on a greater influence over sexual feelings and behaviors. I have seen this happen especially for women in menopause. When their hormone levels dip, the impact of psychological issues such as resentment, anxiety, and past trauma interferes with the motivation and interest in being sexual.

"Saving" Her Sexual Energy for Him?

Selby's distress was not due to her own sense of loss regarding her absent desire; rather, her distress was related to her feeling that she was letting Ethan down. This concern for Ethan's needs and her lack of concern for her own led to her failed strategy of saving what sexual energy she had for Ethan (instead of masturbating when she felt the urge to do so). Historically, sexual desire has been understood as a drive, an innate motivating force that propels one toward satisfaction—in other words, toward sex (be it partnered sex or masturbation). Like hunger or thirst, deprivation is presumed to build energy behind the drive until such a point that the deprived person is compelled to seek out sexual gratification (if you are hungry enough, you will eat). This deprivation strategy is used (mostly unsuccessfully) by many people struggling with low desire, and it is also used by their unhappy partners. However, as we learned in Chapter 1, incentives rather than deprivation motivate sexual desire.

Selby had not masturbated since she began her relationship with Ethan. She felt too guilty: "It's almost as if I were cheating on him." She could not justify using what sexual energy she had for herself. However, this masturbation/deprivation strategy did nothing to improve her desire for sex with Ethan. And by not masturbating, Selby was blocking a pathway for exploring and enjoying her sexuality.

In my work with Selby, I encouraged her to explore the possibility that there was nothing fundamentally flawed about her. I suggested that she consider whether her lack of desire for Ethan meant that something was out of balance—in her life, her relationship, or her way of approaching her relationship with Ethan. As the shame of being a cold (frigid) woman subsided, Selby filled in the blanks in her story, discussing how she had long felt that she needed to be responsible sexually. There could be no room for mistakes, no pregnancies, no sexually transmitted infections, and no bad boyfriends. And while she had sexual desires, she sacrificed desire for responsibility.

ME: Selby, why don't you think you deserve to have pleasure?

SELBY: Oh, but I do. It's just that I need to know that everyone else is okay first.

ME: Oh, I see. Has that ever happened? I mean, have you ever felt that everyone else was okay, or okay enough for you to let your guard down and have fun?

SELBY: Well, not yet. (*pauses*) I see what you're getting at, but Mom and Dad would die if I ever got into trouble. It's bad enough that my brother's in jail, and my sister just doesn't seem to care.

ME: What worries you about the things that might be fun for you? Are they dangerous things? Criminal?

SELBY: Oh, God, no. I just worry that I'm attracted to the wrong type of guy. And before you say anything—it is a real problem. Since I can't seem to say no about anything to anybody, I would be in real trouble if I picked the wrong guy.

ME: Mr. Right sounds a bit boring.

SELBY: Well, yes, actually. I've never really said this out loud, but Ethan is boring.

ME: So, Ethan is safe but boring. (*Selby nods.*) If you could trust yourself a bit more, and trust that you would say no to things you really don't think are okay for you, then maybe life could be a bit more fun?

Paradoxically, Selby and I worked on her saying no rather than on continuing to push her to say yes to sex she did not want to have. We worked on this not just in her sexual relationship but also in her job, her way of dealing with her mother's addiction, her relationship with her sister, and her friendship group. As Selby made gains in therapy, Ethan disappeared. He did not like the new Selby, the Selby who said no. He actually did want to be taken care of; he also wanted to be agreed with and did not want to be challenged. Working with one member of a couple in individual therapy will necessarily affect the relationship dynamic. It is not always destabilizing or relationship ending as it was for Selby and Ethan; it may often lead to growth and positive changes in the other partner and in the relationship. Selby was sad about losing Ethan but recognized that her sense of loss was primarily about what she wished the relationship with Ethan would have been, rather than what it actually was.

Selby eventually transferred from the management side of her marketing firm to the creative team. Instead of yearning for a long-term commitment, Selby decided to have some (responsible) fun in her 30s. Her plan was to date so she could have fun and enjoy herself in a relationship. She also hoped to explore her sexual feelings without the pressure she felt in a committed relationship. Selby was committed to being responsible for herself. She was learning how not to be overly responsible for her partners. She was learning how to be comfortable in her own sexuality. She was learning to trust herself.

If someone feels that they have to have sex, as Selby did, there is no reason to even consider desire. Obligatory sex does not encourage or require sexual desire. And this leads us to Grant.

THE COVER-UP

Grant came to therapy to fulfill a promise he made to his wife, Valerie. Finally finished with his MBA, and with their only child happily into the toddler years, everything seemed perfect except their sex life, which followed a predictable pattern: After several weeks with no sex, Valerie would raise the topic with Grant: "When do you think we can have sex?" He would hear this as both a reasonable request for sex and a complaint. He would respond as if it were the former, staving off his resentment of feeling criticized, and then he would make a date for sex, which he would dutifully perform. After several years of this lackluster routine, Valerie told Grant he needed to get help. While he agreed that the problem was his, he wished that Valerie would have instead considered all the ways in which he was a good, if not ideal, husband and would settle for an infrequent and mediocre sex life. He recognized, however, that Valerie's request was valid, and he made an appointment.

For a man with low desire, Grant actually had a lot of sex, but mostly, he had sex with himself. Grant masturbated regularly, the way one might exercise or load the dishwasher. It was a routine. Typically, in the morning after Valerie left for work, Grant would put on some porn, masturbate, shower, grab a coffee, and head off to the office himself. This ritual took about 45 minutes, with showering and making coffee taking up the bulk of the time. Why was Grant masturbating instead of having sex with Valerie?

ME: You masturbate daily, but that routine doesn't feel driven by desire.

GRANT: That's because it's not.

ME: When do you feel desire?

GRANT: When do I feel horny? Never really. I never really do.

ME: So what happens when you have a date with Valerie for sex?

GRANT: Well, I don't feel horny if that's what you mean. I actually feel really nervous.

ME: Can you tell me more about that?

GRANT: I don't know what there is to tell. If our "date" is at 7, all day long I'm thinking about it. I get a knot in my stomach and feel a bit sick. But I go through with it. I'm not that guy.

ME: That guy?

GRANT: Someone who breaks promises.

Grant told me that he never really lusts and cannot recall a time he did (interestingly, unlike Selby, he did not even consider whether he might be asexual). In high school, he was a self-professed nerd whose free time was spent as a member of the robotics club. He was scrawny and flew under the radar socially. College was a different story. In the summer between high school and college, Grant started to exercise and lift weights because he did not want to look like or be a nerd anymore. In his freshman year of college, he was unprepared for social life. According to Grant, "All my girlfriends were crazy."

ME: Crazy how?

GRANT: They just wanted me to do whatever they wanted to do.

ME: Sexually . . .?

GRANT: Sexually, everything, everything, whatever.

ME: And how did you respond?

GRANT: I just did it.

ME: Sex and everything?

GRANT: (*laughing*) Ya. Sex and everything. I didn't want to be that guy.

ME: The guy that breaks promises.

GRANT: Right! You get it. I don't want to be the guy that hurts people's feelings. The guy that doesn't care. The jerk.

Grant clearly had an overdeveloped sense of responsibility. To him, a relationship was a promise to do whatever the other person wanted. He felt that he could not say no, if saying no hurt someone's feelings or disappointed them. But unlike Selby, who suppressed her sexuality, Grant avoided only partnered sex. He masturbated because he could be sexual without the responsibility he would otherwise feel toward a partner. He did it every day, almost without fail. He was not picky about porn. He just clicked on whatever grabbed his interest—and he masturbated without giving it too much more thought. Grant thought he was an ideal husband in every way except for sex, because he did whatever Valerie wanted and asked of him, no matter how "crazy" it was. But sex with his wife made him anxious. He was anxious about it all day. It was the one thing she asked of him that he could not just mindlessly do. In this way, sex revealed a hidden dynamic: Grant's anxiety about having his own needs in a relationship.

Round Up the Usual Suspects: Testing Testosterone

Many will recognize the above quote from the movie *Casablanca* (Curtiz, 1942; spoiler alert if you have not seen it). Although Rick (Humphrey Bogart) held the still-smoking gun in his hand while the Nazi commander lay slumped on the ground, Captain Renault (Claude Rains) instructed his men to seek the shooter elsewhere: "Major Strasser has been shot. Round up the usual suspects" (Curtiz, 1942, 1:36:45). Even when there is depression, poor body image, relationship turmoil, or other sexual problems that would more than account for low desire, most men will want to find out whether, really, low testosterone is to blame, and most therapists will either endorse their patients' decision or suggest that approach themselves. And why not? Testosterone is widely known as the hormone of desire. It is the usual suspect. And all it takes is a simple blood test. What is the harm?

Ruling out physiological reasons for sexual problems is important (you can refer back to Chapter 2 on this point), and sometimes low testosterone can account for low desire. But unless there is clinically low testosterone (a condition known as hypogonadism), there is simply no data to confirm a relationship between normal levels of testosterone and sexual desire in healthy men or women (van Anders, 2012). Prescribing testosterone to a healthy man may create an expectation of improvement without any other changes being made in lifestyle, mental health, and relationship satisfaction—factors that are more likely to be responsible for low desire. Grant knew that his testosterone was not to blame for his lack of sexual interest in Valerie. For Grant, using testosterone would have just created more pressure. A prescription for testosterone to boost desire in the absence of clinically low levels feeds into the myth that men should be ready, willing, and able to have sex when it is on offer. This erroneous belief in hormonally driven male desire is evident in this quote attributed to comedian Billy Crystal: "Women need a reason to have sex, men just need a place" (Underwood, 1991, 00:07:30). But this myth is responsible for many men finding themselves unable to get an erection in situations in which they think they should (e.g., when there is a willing partner).

We can think back to Luis in Chapter 3. I ask men who are encountering problems getting erections, "Were you interested in having sex?" "Were you turned on?" And when the answer is "no," or "not really," then their expectation for penile performance is the problem, not the performance of the penis. The penis is just doing what it should be doing when it is not aroused—it's just hanging around, waiting, perhaps, for something to happen. In his provocative book *The Existential Importance of the Penis* (Watter, 2023), longtime sex therapist Dan Watter illustrates the problems that can occur when a man fails to understand that his penis has a wisdom of its own. When it does not perform as expected, the penis may be relaying an important message: "I'm not interested," "I'm tired," "I'm channeling your anger," or "I'm hurt."

Grant was actually able to achieve an erection without requiring much stimulation, which is not really the good fortune one might assume. Whether this was an inherent physiological ability or whether it was acquired through years of quick, friction-driven masturbation, Grant's ability to achieve an erection without much mental or emotional arousal allowed him to get by with the dutiful and lackluster partnered sex he had been experiencing for years.

That there is not a direct relationship between hormones and sexuality in men and women is further highlighted by examining the impact of gender-affirming hormone therapy in transgender people. *Transgender* (or *trans*) refers to individuals whose identity does not correspond with the gender assigned at birth. *Transfeminine* describes individuals assigned male at birth who identify as more feminine than masculine, and *transmasculine* describes individuals assigned female at birth who identify as more masculine than feminine. Gender-affirming hormone therapy typically results in greater sexual satisfaction for both transmasculine and transfeminine individuals, despite the fact that testosterone is increased for the former and decreased for the latter. Transmasculine individuals often experience a marked and welcome increase in sexual desire once they start taking testosterone. But despite having reduced levels of testosterone, the increase in sexual frequency and satisfaction experienced by transfeminine individuals demonstrates quite vividly that for almost everyone—transgender, cisgender, and nonbinary—sexual desire needs to be experienced as a positive and pleasurable sensation congruent with one's identity (Ross et al., 2024).

Hungry for Sex?

Valerie was told by her individual therapist, "Relax. Stop initiating sex. Surely Grant will initiate when he feels the desire. Perhaps you are inhibiting Grant by asking for sex too often?" This misguided advice is based on that outdated understanding of sexual desire as a drive. What actually happened when Valerie stopped initiating was that she and Grant stopped having sex—even infrequently. When Valerie told Grant that she was not going to initiate any longer and that she was tired of being rejected, Grant felt sad and guilty (he did not want to reject Valerie), and he felt pressured and confused; without Valerie asking for sex, Grant had no idea how to motivate himself to initiate sex with her. I would have advised Valerie's therapist not to suggest this strategy unless there was also a plan in place for the resumption of sex. The longer couples go without sex, the harder it is for them to find their way back to each other. Although giving Valerie permission to stop initiating sex because it was hurtful to her could create an opening for her to explore her own sexuality in individual therapy, the strategy was not helpful for improving or increasing Grant's sexual desire for Valerie. As advice to Valerie to stop engaging in behavior that is hurting her, and to examine why she continued to do that, it may have been a valuable suggestion indeed.

Far from satiating a couple, good sex leads to a desire for more sex. People who enjoy having sex have it more frequently (McNulty et al., 2016). This also applies to masturbation (Fischer & Træen, 2022). "Saving it"—in other words, not masturbating so you will have energy for your partner—makes sense only if the time frame is short (although there is a high degree of variability—this short time frame can range from a few hours for young and healthy individuals to a few days or more for older individuals [60 and over]).

The Importance of Masturbation

Grant did not know whether Valerie masturbated. He hoped she did, as it would make him feel less guilty. For couples with satisfactory sex lives, masturbation can provide a sexual outlet for times when a partner is not available or interested. Perhaps Valerie had adopted this strategy, but masturbation does not replace partnered sex. Grant did not really know what to think about his daily routine of masturbation. He felt that it likely had no impact on his (absent) desire for sex with Valerie, and it certainly had no impact on his ability to perform the dutiful sex he had with her on a bimonthly basis.

Masturbation can be a wonderful way to discover and uncover one's sexuality. It can provide an opportunity to engage in behaviors and enjoy fantasies that one may not want to entertain in reality or with a partner. Grant and Selby were using masturbation in opposite ways to the same end: to avoid their own sexual desires. Grant masturbated so that he would not feel desire, while Selby, who did not masturbate, avoided knowing and enjoying her desires. This is the tricky aspect of talking about sex in psychotherapy: You cannot just ask about masturbation (or any other sexual behavior) and know what the answer means. You have to ask follow-up questions and risk feeling the discomfort of being perceived as intrusive or naive. Consider this interaction I had early on in therapy with Grant (and as you are reading, know that the tone is friendly, calm, a bit jokey at times, and always, on my part, nonjudgmental and reassuring). Initially, Grant was taken aback by the detailed nature of the questions and was mildly defensive.

ME: So how often do you masturbate? (Note that I take my own advice from Chapter 2 and assume he masturbates—he can correct me if he does not.)

GRANT: (*nervous laughter*) Really? We're going to go there?

ME: Yup. We're going to go there. (I do not need to justify the question.)

GRANT: I don't know. I don't count. The normal amount, I guess.

ME: So . . . several times a day or once a year on your birthday? (I give what I think is an exaggerated estimate of normal so that Grant can feel comfortable with whatever he answers.)

GRANT: (*laughs in relief*) Not several times a day. Usually once a day, sometimes twice.

ME: Okay. So, what prompts you to masturbate once or twice a day?

GRANT: I don't know. I just feel like it, I guess. Why does anyone masturbate?

ME: You feel like it . . . so you feel like having sexual pleasure? (I do not take the bait proffered in the second part of his answer as his question is really meant to deflect.)

GRANT: I guess. I masturbate in the morning just as a routine. It's just something I do, like before I get dressed—I jerk off.

ME: Okay, so masturbating is part of your morning routine. (*Grant nods.*) And what makes you masturbate another time, when you masturbate twice a day?

GRANT: Oh, that is usually because I want to go to sleep.

ME: Okay, got it. Once a day is part of your routine, and sometimes twice if you need help going to sleep. (*Grant nods.*) So, how do you masturbate? Do you always use porn? Do you fantasize?

GRANT: Isn't this TMI [too much information]?

ME: Grant, there's really no TMI in therapy.

GRANT: (*laughs*) Okay, fair enough. In the morning, it's porn. And at night it's usually just the friction that does it. I'm not thinking of anything or anyone; I'm not wishing I was with someone other than Valerie if that's what you're getting at.

ME: What about the porn? How do you choose? (Again, I do not get deflected by Grant.)

GRANT: Whatever their algorithm is on me, I go with it. I just click on whatever is suggested. I don't have the time to browse around. Naked women and men having sex. That's all I need.

Grant tries to put me off by telling me that he masturbates a "normal" amount and that the reason he masturbates is the same reason that everyone masturbates. He invites me to make assumptions so he does not need to risk revealing himself to me. But I do take the necessary risk of being seen as naive or even stupid by persevering with my questions. Grant likely felt defensive about his daily masturbation to porn; he does not want to be judged. But if I had responded, "Oh, the normal amount—so once or twice a week?" I doubt he would have corrected me, and there would have been a lot I would not have known. I can also take the risk of being experienced as intrusive because I know why I am asking about masturbation: It helps me understand how he approaches sexuality and his relationships more fully. I am not simply curious.

Grant's family history, as with all family histories, was important for understanding his sexual dilemma. Grant's mother was an anxious and emotionally fragile person, and his father was verbally and emotionally abusive to her and to Grant (an only child). Grant grew up feeling angry at his mother for being weak, yet he felt compelled to compensate for his father's behavior. As Grant described it in our first meeting, "I really can't stand my mother, but I'd do anything for her." The disconnect between his emotions and his behavior was already set.

So, during his college years, Grant continued this pattern of doing "sex and everything" for a series of "crazy girlfriends." In other words, he continued this pattern of ignoring his feelings in order to be a dutiful boyfriend. Whether these girlfriends were indeed "crazy," I will not ever know, but the dynamic Grant described clearly was. He felt that he needed to do whatever his girlfriends asked of him. This included engaging in not only unwanted social obligations but also sexual obligations. For example, Grant felt obliged to have sex with two women simultaneously when he was still unsure of whether he could sexually satisfy one, and he agreed to and had sex multiple times in one day with his girlfriend, which was several times more than he had any interest in. He was a lucky guy—right? According to cultural stereotypes, what man would not want to have a threesome and a sexually insatiable and drop-dead-gorgeous girlfriend? But Grant did not feel like a lucky guy. The pattern that was set in childhood was extended to his sexuality. Even years later, Grant found that the only times he could truly enjoy sex was when he was by himself.

The pattern of subjugating his own feelings to satisfy the needs of others resonated strongly with Grant. He started to notice all the ways that pattern played out in his life: Grant never knew when a work request was reasonable or not, so he often found himself working late and on weekends when others in his group were not doing the same. He never had parties because he never knew how to set a limit on guests. And when his uncle offered to teach him to play tennis, Grant bought three new racquets because he did not want to show up with the wrong equipment (and he actually had little interest in learning to play). Grant felt that he needed to meet whatever the expectations were of him; to do otherwise caused him tremendous anxiety. As he worked in therapy to be more assertive at work and to set better boundaries with his mother, his friends, and Valerie, he started to have panic attacks and back pain. These concerning symptoms required targeted treatment interventions (breathing, relaxation, cognitive restructuring), and eventually Grant was better able to both manage his anxiety and set better boundaries.

But sex was resistant to change. Grant continued to find it incredibly difficult to be sexual with Valerie. "I just don't want to" was the refrain in his head, and his body would only respond during sex if he closed his eyes and concentrated on himself. He was tuning Valerie out, and rather than finding her pleasure and desires arousing, to him they were stressful demands.

Not wanting to have sex with Valerie was the symptom that brought Grant to therapy, but underneath that was a man who found relating to others very stressful. The therapy relationship was a revelation to him in that it was the first time he did not have to stress about someone else's needs and expectations (although he struggled with this in the beginning). The paradox of not wanting to disappoint Valerie and yet routinely disappointing her (not desiring her) was revisited many times. Always in therapy, though, we returned to Grant—his feelings, his desires, and his bodily reactions—so he could stop the pattern of ignoring his own feelings. On his own initiative, Grant tried the experiment of forgoing masturbation. It did not have the hoped-for effect of increasing his desire for Valerie (or any other person), but it did illuminate for him how dependent he was on masturbation as a way to regulate his mood and calm his anxiety. Grant did find it helpful to refrain from masturbating for a few days prior to his "date" for sex with Valerie, in terms of being able to reach orgasm.

At the time of this writing, Grant remains in therapy. He has sex with Valerie about twice a month—as often as he did before he started therapy. The difference is that he is present during sex with Valerie and more focused on pleasure than performance. He still feels selfish when he is focused on his own pleasure, and he still gets slightly anxious when he focuses on Valerie's arousal and enjoyment, but he is getting there.

SEX ROLES, GENDER STEREOTYPES, AND A DIFFERENT MEASURE OF DESIRE

Selby and Grant presented with similar issues: a lack of desire for partners they care about. But in many respects, they differed significantly, as with their masturbation habits. One factor to consider is that these two patients differed because of gender roles. Exploring the impact of cultural, societal, and familial expectations can offer our patients the opportunity to look at themselves through a different lens: "what shaped me" rather than "what's wrong with me." Like many of the therapeutic techniques and strategies described in this book, offering different perspectives and examining the impact of sociocultural and family of origin influences is part of our skill set as therapists. The fact that the topic is sex does not change that.

Grant knew that Valerie was distraught not only because he did not want sex but also because she wanted sex more than Grant did. "It's not supposed to be that way," Valerie told him. It took Valerie a long time to ask Grant to go to therapy because, for a very long time, she attributed his lack of desire to her concern that she was not desirable. The belief, previously discussed, that men's sex drive is biologically driven can lead to erroneous conclusions like Valerie's ("I'm not desirable") and may lead men, like Grant, to have unreasonable expectations for their desire ("I should want sex no matter what"). In fact, this belief that men are, or should be, ready, willing, and able to have sex whenever it is offered led Grant to have a lot of sex during his college years that he never wanted. In the same way that Grant did a lot of things he did not want to do, he obliged sexually, and his own sexual desires went unexplored and ignored.

Selby believed, as Valerie did, that men want sex more than women do, so Selby felt that it was natural for Ethan to want and need to have more sex than she did. Selby focused on Ethan's need for sex, rather than his desire for a sexual connection with her. But she also felt that if she loved Ethan, she should want to have sex with him, conflating love with sexual desire and buying into the stereotyped notion that men want sex and women want love.

There is truth regarding an imbalance in levels of sexual desire between men and women, but as with many truths, the reality is more complex. Recent research from a large-scale, longitudinal Finnish study found that when measured quantitatively (frequency of sexual behavior), men's sexual desire is typically higher than women's (Harris et al., 2023). But problems with low desire are not uncommon for either gender. Meta-analyses of prevalence studies show that a third of women report problems with low desire in relationships, with that figure rising to 54% of postmenopausal women (Khani et al., 2021). Estimates of low sexual desire in men also show increased problems as men age, and depending on methodology, prevalence rates fall between 14% and 41% (G. A. Wang et al., 2023). In addition to age, other factors affect sexual desire. The authors of the Finnish study concluded that "men, just like women, fluctuate in the degree to which they desire sex, and are equally impacted by general affective states (such as how stressed they feel) and a number of relationship-oriented states (such as how close they feel to their partner)" (Harris et al., 2023, p. 1476). So, qualitatively speaking, men and women are not so different in their experience of sexual desire after all.

Gendered stereotypes of desire are blatantly evident in same-sex relationships (e.g., the stereotypes of the hypersexual gay man and the nonsexual lesbian). The belief that gay men engage in a lot of (risky) sex with a lot of different men (in other words, gay men are "promiscuous") is a belief often endorsed by the lay public, as well as by scientists and clinicians (Nimbi et al., 2020). Research on risk regarding HIV and other sexually transmitted infections tends to validate this stereotype and disregards the reality of diversity within the gay community. But studies have shown that low sexual desire can be a frequent complaint for gay men in relationships, with estimates ranging between 8% and a shocking 57% (Nimbi et al., 2020). One study found that low desire in gay men was related to their fear of not performing well sexually, a concern that heterosexual men shared, but not to the same degree (Kowalczyk et al., 2017). And while daily stress reduced sexual interest for gay men in long-term relationships, emotional closeness and a desire for validation provided a buffer from these negative effects and increased motivation for intimate partnered sex (Bancroft et al., 2003; Hiemstra et al., 2024). The stereotype of the promiscuous gay man masks important emotional issues and influences on their sexual interest.

On the other end of the stereotyping spectrum, there is "lesbian bed death," a term used to refer to the purported drop in sexual frequency experienced by women in committed same-sex relationships (Frederick et al., 2021). Closer examination reveals that far from giving up on sex, many lesbians may simply do sex differently. While the frequency of sexual interactions is often reported to be lower among lesbian couples than heterosexuals, lesbians report experiencing more consistent orgasms, engaging in mutual oral sex more frequently, and in general, having more sexual variety, including using sex toys. Their sexual encounters take time—most were more than half an hour, with some lasting over an hour. The time and effort, as well as the expectations of intimacy and reciprocity, may surely make it difficult to have many "quickies." Quality, not quantity, may make for a better measure of life in the lesbian bed. I would argue that quality surpasses quantity as a measure of sexual happiness for a diverse and wide range of people of all sexual orientations.

DESIRE IS THE REAL ORGASM

Selby and Grant were distressed not only because their partners wanted to have more frequent sex but also because they were aware that "just doing it" would not suffice. As Ethan said to Selby, "I don't want to have to beg or insist; I just want you to want me." It was not enough to agree to sex; the request from their partners was to desire them sexually.

In a *New York Times Magazine* feature article, Marta Meana, a sex researcher from the University of Nevada, Las Vegas, summed it up thus: "Being desired is the orgasm" (Bergner, 2009, para. 36). This phrase resonated with a lot of people; several major news outlets picked up the story, and Meana found herself on *The Oprah Winfrey Show*, a wildly popular daytime talk show. On the show, Meana clarified that the anticipation and buildup to sexual pleasure is what really excites and motivates women: "I'm not knocking orgasms. . . . But being desired is extremely arousing for women. The reason for that is that being desired means that a man doesn't just want to have sex. He wants to have sex with *you*" ("Sexual Desire: The Real Female Orgasm," 2009). Although Meana's research was focused on women (Meana, 2010), something similar is at work in men's psyches. Many of my male patients have echoed Ethan's desire to be desired, and research studies confirm that this is true for a majority of men (Murray et al., 2017). For many men and women, the real satisfaction from sex comes from desire: anticipation and the feeling of being wanted. So, the absence of desire is a very big absence indeed.

Wanting to feel desired by your partner is different from being objectified or sexualized by others. Objectification is a dehumanizing experience sadly familiar to many people, especially women, and particularly Asian women and people of color (Cheeseborough et al., 2020). Transgender and nonbinary individuals report depersonalizing experiences of being fetishized (Anzani et al., 2021). Statements such as "I was being talked to as if I were a sex toy" (Anzani et al., 2021, p. 904) summarize their feelings. Others had more ambivalence: "When having practically no option for feeling desired, being fetishized seems better than having no attention at all" and "I'm into kink so it's usually fine" (Anzani et al., 2021, p. 906).

Selby, like many others who have low desire, experienced her partner's interest in her as objectification. Ethan's sexual overtures were received not with pleasure but with dread.

Selby was disconnected from her own sense of sexual agency. To Selby, there was no difference between being whistled at by a group of rowdy drunks and being flirted with by an interesting and interested man, or for that matter being approached by her lover.

UNDERSTANDING THE PLIGHT OF THE HIGHER-DESIRING PARTNER

When reading the brief case descriptions, some of you might notice that your sympathies differ for the undesired partners. You may feel sympathetic toward Valerie, and you may feel annoyed with Ethan. I have portrayed these partners to you in the way they were portrayed to me by my patients. I did not ever meet Valerie or Ethan.

We need to remember that sometimes our patients are unreliable narrators of their own lives, as their understanding of their experiences may be distorted by their own psychological issues. It was easy to understand why Grant married Valerie. He told me that she not only was a kind and loving partner but also did not ask for much. It was not as easy, therefore, to understand why Grant did not want to have sex with Valerie. Selby portrayed Ethan as demanding, childish, and needy, so it was easy to understand why she would not want to have sex with him.

The pitfall for therapists is blaming the partner; in my case, the pitfall would be thinking that Selby's problems would be solved if she ditched Ethan. I had to be conscious of maintaining a therapeutic detachment so I could acknowledge, understand, and empathize with Grant and Selby while being aware that there are other ways of viewing their situations. Grant's view of Valerie reinforced his feelings of guilt and obligation. If I focused my efforts on helping Grant be sexual with his kind and deserving wife, I would be adding to the pressure he already felt. Instead, I needed to work with

Grant on reexamining the level of obligation he felt in relationships. Valerie may be, as Grant portrayed her, kind and deserving, but perhaps she was also a bit more resilient. Perhaps she had some agency too. Selby wanted to have a relationship with Ethan and twisted herself into a pretzel to please him. Was Ethan really as childishly needy as Selby perceived him to be? Or perhaps all she really knew was how to relate to someone's needs.

Higher-desiring partners are not always, or even often, just selfish people who only want sex. I frequently challenge my patients on this point, as I challenged Selby with this question: "If Ethan only wants sex, why does he stay with you? It seems like sex is quite easy to get, so why would Ethan choose to be with you when you don't have a lot of interest in having sex?" This challenge helped Selby consider whether Ethan's desire to have a sexual relationship with her was a genuine desire for an intimate connection and a wish to be seen as desirable. This question helped Selby understand that it is she, not Ethan, who sees sex as an obligation to be fulfilled rather than a pleasure to share and enjoy.

WHY NOT DO COUPLES THERAPY?

As you are reading these cases, you may wonder why I did not suggest inviting the patients' partners to participate in therapy. The issue of whether to see an individual or a couple is an important clinical consideration, so let me share my thoughts on this subject as it pertains to Selby and Grant.

Sex is contextual, and almost invariably, people come to therapy for sexual issues that are relational in nature. Grant's solo sex was in reaction to how stressful he found it to be sexual with Valerie (or anyone). Many of Grant's issues revolved around Valerie's "demands" and on the fact that he was not attracted to her or aroused by her during sex. It would have been incredibly hurtful to Valerie to hear these things, and Grant needed to be able to talk about them and process them in therapy. Knowing Valerie only through Grant reflected what was essential to him about their relationship and the expectations he had of himself in relationships.

The fact that Grant's view of Valerie changed over time revealed his treatment progress. At first, Valerie was demanding and a bit crazy. She asked for inexplicable things that he felt compelled to do—such as move her desk a few feet to a sunnier area of the study (not an easy task), go on walks when it was clearly going to rain (Crazy—doesn't she look at the weather?), or preserve their son's baby clothes in a memory box (Donate them! There is no storage room in our house!). Initially, what Grant talked about in therapy mirrored his perceptions of a demanding and crazy wife whom he needed to appease and that his pleasure must be solo. Then, as Grant felt less obliged to please others, his perceptions changed: Valerie was less crazy and more sentimental. If Grant did not feel desire, he at least felt more open to having sex with his sentimental and reasonable wife. As their sex life improved and as Grant's boundaries with others improved, his sexual relationship with Valerie also improved, and this interdependent cycle slowly wound its way to a better overall resolution. Had Valerie been in therapy with him, Grant would have retreated, would likely have been guided by what he thought Valerie wanted him to say, and would not have been able to explore his feelings about sex as openly as he did.

A similar logic was at play in my decision not to invite Ethan into therapy. Selby would not have been able to be as open in exploring her own thoughts, feelings, and behaviors in relation to Ethan if he had been present. But of course, I could have witnessed this dynamic had both been present. Importantly, Selby had an ambivalent commitment to her relationship, and she wanted to do therapy on her own. (You can skip ahead to Chapter 8 for a discussion of working with couples on desire issues.)

MEDICATIONS WITH SEXUAL SIDE EFFECTS

By now, most of us are familiar with the sexual side effects associated with many antidepressant medications. Reported side effects include loss of sexual interest, difficulty experiencing orgasm (takes a long time or the sensation of orgasm may be diminished) as well as arousal problems (including erectile dysfunction). Because sexual dysfunction is often a symptom of anxiety or depression, it is sometimes difficult to attribute sexual problems to the medications used to treat these conditions. Their culpability is clear, however, when the sexual problems coincide with the initiation of the medication. Selective serotonin reuptake inhibitors (SSRIs), serotonin–norepinephrine reuptake inhibitors (SNRIs), and the tricyclic clomipramine are considered to be high risk for the development of sexual side effects. Some estimates suggest that as many as 80% of people taking one or more of these medications will develop sexual side effects, with fewer patients reporting sexual problems unless specifically asked (Rothmore, 2020). Also quite alarming is the fact that since 2006, there have been credible reports in the medical literature of SSRI-induced sexual dysfunction persisting after the medication is no longer being taken. Sexual side effects are also reported for antipsychotic medications, and as with the antidepressants, unwanted sexual side effects are a leading cause of noncompliance with medication protocols (Montejo et al., 2021; Rothmore, 2020).

Educating patients about the risks of sexual side effects associated with medication is important, even when sexual issues are not part of their presenting complaint. But it is imperative to discuss sexual side effects when sex is already problematic. Prescribers can offer lower doses, switch medications, or suggest medication holidays; therapists can be supportive and encouraging of patients, as they may need to make changes in their sexual activities to increase stimulation.

SUMMARY

This chapter explored the struggles that people experience when desire is divorced from sex. Two cases highlighted an important but often neglected aspect of encountering desire problems in psychotherapy: the damaging effect of seeing sex as a duty or obligation. Many patients with low desire, along with their partners, expect therapists to encourage them to be sexual. Sometimes they expect the therapist to uncover their inherent and fundamental psychic flaw that has inhibited their desire. Other times, they hope that the therapist has some intervention or suggestion that will quickly make sex desirable. But there really is nothing sexy about obligatory sex. Obligation is the enemy of desire.

Understanding that sexual desire can mirror and often magnify psychological dynamics can be helpful when patients present with desire problems. The cases in this chapter demonstrated how desire problems can magnify psychological issues (Grant's anxiety related to having needs in a relationship) and how issues in other areas of functioning can provide insight into desire problems (Selby's need to manage relationships). Instead of contributing to the pressure patients feel to have sex, therapy can instead help patients who struggle with desire to set boundaries, to say no instead of always feeling they must say yes, and to make room to explore their own desire without the pressure to feel something they do not.

If desire is the real orgasm, obligatory sex will never do.

6 WORKING WITH SURVIVORS OF CHILDHOOD SEXUAL ABUSE

Surviving is defined in the Oxford Languages (n.d.) dictionary as "continuing to exist; remaining intact." Survivors of sexual abuse may well question the applicability of this word as it applies to them. The understanding that surviving is a process may be appreciated, but many survivors do not feel intact. When they look in the metaphoric mirror, they see, first and foremost, the cracks, the fault lines, if you will. Many survivors say and feel that they are barely holding it together. So, we must understand that psychotherapy is a risky proposition for survivors. They have spent much of their lives trying to distance themselves from their abuse, and they are reluctant, at best, to relive it in therapy. They are afraid of falling apart. Many of them are also afraid that others, therapists included, will see what they see when they look in the mirror: that the cracks are, in fact, fault lines, and the fault is theirs.

Survivors need a reason to go to therapy, and the hope of having meaningful relationships with a satisfying sex life is one such reason. This chapter reviews research on the effects of sexual abuse and then focuses on the sensitivity and skills needed to engage in the therapeutic process of helping survivors have positive sexual experiences. First, let me introduce you to Jessica and Daniel, two survivors who were motivated to seek therapy after years of

https://doi.org/10.1037/0000483-007
Talking About Sex in Psychotherapy: A Guide for Every Therapist, by K. S. K. Hall

silence by a desire to have more fulfilling sex lives. Their therapies illustrate many of the core treatment processes outlined in this chapter.

Jessica, a first-generation Korean American woman, came to therapy prepared to talk about the sexual abuse she suffered from a physician. Jessica hoped she would not have to talk about her history of being sexually abused by her father from ages 7 to 10. She was 29 years old when she came to therapy for the first time, almost 2 decades after the fact. Jessica believed that she was unlovable; she thought this belief was both the reason for and the result of the incest. Jessica had held herself together, successfully avoiding triggers for her posttraumatic stress disorder (PTSD) until she was in a relationship. Finally, with someone she loved, flashbacks threatened her ability to have sex. Jessica came to therapy when her fear of losing her partner outweighed her fear of talking about the past.

Daniel had been in therapy several times before, but only briefly, before staying in therapy with me for years. He was willing to try therapy again because he was desperate to get his sexual behavior under control. Despite his best intentions, he kept cracking along the usual fault lines: Being overcome with anxiety until having sex with sex workers somehow made him feel that he could continue to keep himself together. Daniel stayed in therapy and talked about the sexual abuse he thought he would keep secret, because this time in therapy, he made the connection from the past to his present problems.

EFFECTS OF CHILDHOOD SEXUAL ABUSE

Both the empirical literature and clinical experience indicate that sexual abuse can result in various negative outcomes related to sex for both men and women. Many survivors can engage in sex (e.g., function) but have trouble enjoying sex. So, despite experiencing pain or anxiety or outright fear, and despite dissociation and flashbacks, many survivors do what they learned to do in childhood: They endure.

Effects on Women

Between 65% and 85% of women with histories of child sexual abuse (CSA) report experiencing sexual problems, which is an alarming statistic (Pulverman & Meston, 2020). During the many years of my practice with survivors in individual, couples, and group therapy, I have had the privilege of being trusted with many stories of problematic sex: Maggie, who felt she found Mr. Right only to discover that her body screamed "No!" when he approached her sexually; Janine, who could not stand to have her breasts touched and who always wore a bra during sex; Petra, who was repulsed by the sight of her boyfriend's penis; Lily, who was unsure of her sexual orientation; Cara, who had sex with her roommate's boyfriend while her roommate was crying in the next room; June, who could barely utter the word "sex"; and Elizabeth, who watched incest porn. Research affirms the broad spectrum of sexual problems that we see in clinical practice: sexual dysfunctions (low or absent desire, difficulty getting or staying aroused or reaching orgasm, pain or fear of pain during vaginal penetration), sexual revictimization, engaging in risky sexual behaviors (increasing the risk of contracting a sexually transmitted infection [STI] or having an unintended pregnancy), avoiding sex or specific sexual activities, having flashbacks or dissociating during sex, and having intrusive thoughts or sexual fantasies of the abuse (Abu-Raya & Gewirtz-Meydan, 2023; Bigras et al., 2021; Gewirtz-Meydan & Lassri, 2023; Noll, 2021; Pulverman & Meston, 2020).

Emotional reactions such as anxiety, fear, guilt, shame, and disgust can be attached to sex (Pulverman et al., 2018). Pulverman and Meston (2020) found that sexual shame had a unique contribution to the development and maintenance of sexual dysfunctions in survivors. Negative cognitions about sex, and the sexual self of the survivor, such as "I have to have sex to be loved," "I don't deserve sexual pleasure," and "Sex is disgusting," are related to reduced sexual pleasure (Bigras et al., 2021). Negative cognitions can reinforce shame and guilt, and can contribute to relationship distress (Abu-Raya & Gewirtz-Meydan, 2023), further diminishing sexual pleasure.

Effects on Men

In their review of the small but growing literature on the impact of childhood sexual abuse on the sexual functioning of men, Gewirtz-Meydan and Opuda (2022) reported a wide range in terms of the prevalence of sexual dysfunction—from 12% to 69%. Specific diagnoses for which there were reported rates were erectile dysfunction (33%), hypoactive sexual desire disorder (24%), and premature ejaculation (15%). While these rates do not appear to be significantly different from the rates reported for the general population (see Laumann et al., 1999), survivors may have different reasons or causative factors underlying their sexual problems. Many men with histories of CSA report dissociating during sexual activity; in fact, in one study, over 50% of male survivors seeking therapy reported dissociation during sex (Villeneuve et al., 2024). Since pleasurable and functional sex requires a connection to one's body, dissociation, defined as the feeling of being disconnected from one's physical self, makes it difficult to experience sexual pleasure (Chen et al., 2024) and to know one's needs and wants—a critical element for sexual desire and arousal (Villeneuve et al., 2024).

Historically, research on male survivors' sexuality has focused on the propensity toward hypersexuality, sexual aggression, and risky sexual behaviors rather than on sexual problems that might interfere with the experience of sexual pleasure (Villeneuve et al., 2024). In other words, a great deal of attention has been placed on making sure men do not become abusers when they have a history of sexual abuse. However, the purportedly strong connection between CSA and sex offending or sexual aggression is not so clear and not so strong when looking at studies in the aggregate and accounting for the quality of the research (Hui et al., 2024). What is clear is that the vast majority of boys who are sexually abused do not go on to become men who abuse children or sexually assault women. A history of CSA is only one factor that, when paired with other traumatic life events and substance abuse, can predispose an individual to engage in sexually risky or sexually aggressive behavior (Hui et al., 2024; Noll, 2021; Peterson et al., 2018).

The myth that boys who are sexually abused will go on to become abusers themselves has had a profound effect on many male survivors, who have been terrified that this will be their fate. I have worked with many male survivors who did not want to disclose their abuse or seek treatment for fear that they would be seen as pedophiles in the making. Many of them had suppressed their sexuality for fear of being attracted to children. Sometimes the distress rose to the level where a diagnosis of obsessive-compulsive disorder (OCD) could be considered.

OCD and Sexual Anxiety

Recurrent, distressing, and intrusive thoughts are a dominant symptom of OCD. Distressing and repugnant sexual thoughts may be part of the symptom complex, and 20% to 30% of individuals (both men and women) with OCD report that their primary obsessional concern deals with such unwanted thoughts (Bonagura et al., 2022). Two common concerns involve worry about sexual orientation (SO-OCD) and worry about pedophilic arousal (P-OCD).

Obsessive worry about pedophilic ideation can be wrongly diagnosed as pedophilia (Bonagura et al., 2022) and can cause enormous stress as well as occupational and relational impairment (Schild et al., 2024). Bruce and colleagues (2018) outlined an assessment and treatment protocol for OCD sufferers who have obsessive thoughts regarding an attraction to children. According to these authors, the important distinction between P-OCD and pedophilia centers on emotional reactions. People with OCD fear that they are attracted to children and fear that they will engage sexually with children.

They often avoid contact with children, even their own, to mitigate the risk. Sexual thoughts regarding children produce anxiety, shame, and disgust. People with P-OCD spend hours worrying about the possibility of an attraction to children. There is no sexual arousal or pleasure that results from these thoughts. This is in contrast to people who are attracted to children, as they are aroused by thoughts of sexual contact with them.

SO-OCD is also characterized by worry and uncertainty. The distress caused by SO-OCD arises from doubt and uncertainty regarding sexual attraction, rather than internalized homophobia, which is characterized by negative reactions to the sexual minority group. In SO-OCD, there is compulsive checking to detect any signs of arousal to the nonpreferred gender (Williams et al., 2015). This also occurs in P-OCD, where the checking centers on genital responses to children. Both SO-OCD and P-OCD result in avoidance of situations in which unwanted arousal may occur (contact with children or with people of the nonpreferred gender). Treatment involving exposure and response prevention, the gold standard for the treatment of OCD, is recommended, and the interested reader is referred to the article by Bruce et al. (2018) as well as a treatment manual for sexual obsessions (Williams & Wetterneck, 2019).

Mechanisms of Sexual Trauma: Multiple Models

Finkelhor and Browne (1985) were the first to propose a model for how childhood sexual abuse can affect women in adulthood. Although the model was based on their research regarding father–daughter incest, it has applicability beyond that group and has been widely applied to both male and female survivors of intra- and extrafamilial sexual abuse (Finkelhor, 1990).

The model highlights four pathways by which sexual abuse can disrupt later adult sexual functioning. Three of the four traumagenic factors (i.e., leading to trauma) are not specific to sexual abuse: betrayal (violation of trust, being manipulated), powerlessness (resulting from exploitation and not being able to protect oneself), and stigmatization (the feeling of being different, damaged by the abuse). These three factors interfere with many of the foundations important to sex: trusting yourself so that you can trust your sexual choices, being able to be vulnerable in the presence of another person, and feeling entitled to pleasure. Survivors of other forms of childhood abuse and neglect may also experience sexual problems in adulthood. Unique to sexual abuse is the traumagenic pathway of traumatic sexualization, which accounts for the impact of early, unwanted, and forced sexual activity on the formation of sexual values, attitudes, and norms. Sexual shame, confusion, and alterations of arousal patterns can also be related to traumatic sexualization.

Briere (1996) offered a developmental perspective to further explain how childhood attachment dynamics and children's cognitive understanding of self, others, and the future are disrupted by abuse and can come to disrupt adult sexuality. According to Briere, the experience of posttraumatic stress in childhood negatively affects subsequent mental and emotional development and fosters a reliance on primitive and inadequate coping mechanisms (denial, dissociation, avoidance). In other words, sexual abuse in childhood, along with the coping mechanisms necessary to deal with it, sends children down a developmental pathway that can lead to problems in adolescence and then adulthood.

MacIntosh (2019) noted that the developmental impact of childhood maltreatment (including nonsexual forms of abuse) can lead to a bifurcated trajectory of either inhibited or disinhibited sexuality. *Disinhibition*—engaging in risky sexual behavior or having a high number of sexual partners (concurrently or sequentially)—can result in STIs, unwanted pregnancy, reputational damage, and self-esteem problems, issues that can have a lasting effect on the trajectory of one's life. Avoidance of sex in adolescence can likewise interfere with developing social and sexual skills, and can lead to self-esteem problems and an isolated lifestyle, problems that are likely to persist into adulthood. Why one person becomes sexually disinhibited and another shuts down sexually is not entirely clear. But it is similar to how some patients manage the dysregulation of PTSD: Some engage in avoidance behaviors, and others, in an attempt at mastery, engage in what appears to be a repetition of the trauma (MacIntosh, 2024). Whether inhibited or disinhibited, the earlier sexual behaviors will, in turn, have an impact on future sexuality.

Based on a meta-analysis and comprehensive literature review, Noll (2021) argued for a model focusing on the additive effect of many factors uniquely inherent in sexual abuse. Called the compounded convergence of mechanisms (CCM) model, Noll (2021) stated that, in addition to the four traumagenic mechanisms in Finkelhor and Browne's (1985) model (betrayal, powerlessness, stigmatization, and traumatic sexualization), CSA survivors have a high likelihood of experiencing additional risk factors, including insecure attachment, avoidance, emotion dysregulation, and the biological embedding of stress. While Noll (2021) found that single factors (e.g., attachment problems) confer relatively low risk for problematic sexual adjustment, risk increases with the co-occurrence and overlap of many traumagenic mechanisms (e.g., negative cognitions, attachment problems, relationship distress, PTSD symptoms). Incorporating the results of accumulated research, the CCM model predicts that experiencing PTSD, anxiety, and traumatic sexualization in childhood are key factors that increase the likelihood of sexual difficulties in adulthood.

INTRODUCING THE SUBJECT OF SEX TO SURVIVORS

Survivors often strain to see what they would have been like, what they would or could have accomplished, had their potential not been shattered by sexual abuse. Survivors are left to wonder about the nature and quality of their current or future relationships if their trust had not been violated at such a young age and if their sexuality had not been distorted by abuse. A chance to reclaim lost potential is a motivating factor for therapy. In cases of CSA, a chance to enjoy sex is a strong motivating factor for therapy. There are several pathways by which CSA is purported to disrupt sexual pleasure, and there are several theories accounting for these multiple effects. Identifying these pathways guides treatment decisions and, when explicit, helps survivors better understand the need to talk about their painful past.

In my training seminars and workshops, therapists have told me that they are hesitant to raise the subject of sex with their survivor patients, despite the knowledge that most, if not all, of their survivor patients will have sexual difficulties. Therapists are worried that talking explicitly about sex will trigger or upset their patients, will be a boundary violation, or will be perceived as such. Therapists are also concerned about bringing up the topic of sex when they are not sure what to do with any issues that may be revealed. Often, they fall back on the pernicious belief in a naturally occurring and universal sexual response, so that once the trauma is healed, good sex will naturally follow. (For those of you who have read the preceding chapters, you have hopefully been disabused of this belief.)

I raise the topic of sex with the groups I lead, the couples I see, and the individuals I treat. In groups for sexual abuse survivors, I introduce the topic by saying that many women who are sexually abused in childhood experience difficulties with sexuality in adulthood. I am purposely vague about what those difficulties might be, and I then ask if this resonates with any of them. It usually just takes one woman in the group to start talking before the others share their own stories. I may offer, at some appropriate point in the discussion, examples of some of the sexual consequences of abuse that are difficult for most women to acknowledge, such as intrusive thoughts of the abuse during sex or masturbation, flashbacks during sex or masturbation, shame, guilt, hypervigilance, and being aroused by thoughts, memories, or fantasies of the sexual abuse, which may trigger orgasm during partnered sex and to which they may masturbate. I do something similar in individual therapy with male and female survivors and in individual sessions in the context of couples therapy. When I introduce the topic of sex, I invite discussion, I may ask more specific questions if the discussion becomes stalled, and I try to ease the shame by offering examples of some of the more difficult sexual problems to acknowledge.

Note that I do not ask about CSA in couples therapy when both partners are present, in case one partner is not aware of the history. When I ask about CSA in sessions with each partner individually, as part of couples therapy, I guarantee confidentiality so that patients will be more likely to disclose if the CSA is a secret. See Chapter 4 regarding secrets in therapy and Chapter 8 on couples therapy for more information.

JESSICA'S STORY

Jessica was reading the newspaper, as she did most mornings. One day, however, while reading a particular article, she had a flashback to the sexual abuse that shattered her equilibrium years ago. The newspaper article that triggered her flashback described the recent conviction of Jessica's former gynecologist on multiple counts of sexual abuse brought by 11 women who were patients in his practice. Jessica had been abused by this physician also, but the flashback she experienced that day pertained to her earlier abuse by her biological father. Jessica contacted me for therapy because my name was mentioned in the newspaper article as the expert witness called by the prosecution. She therefore trusted me, even before meeting me, to believe her. Even prior to that morning when she read the newspaper, Jessica knew she needed to go to therapy because she was experiencing flashbacks during the first consensual sexual relationship she had ever had.

Jessica was experiencing posttraumatic stress symptoms (PTSS) when she was having sex with her partner. Specifically, Jessica had flashbacks, feeling that she was back across time and space and was again being sexually assaulted by her father. At these times, Jessica was no longer having sex with her fiancé, Justin, and she was unable to experience a sensual and emotional connection with her body, her sexuality, and her partner.

Fear was part of Jessica's sexual experiences, making her hypervigilant during sex; she scanned for signs that she would have a flashback, that Justin would know she was not enjoying the sex, or that Justin was not enjoying the sex. All these symptoms were new to Jessica because she had completely avoided partnered sex until she unexpectedly met Justin in her late 20s. Women who experience sex-related PTSS often use avoidance as a coping strategy; they avoid sex altogether, as had Jessica; if they are partnered, they avoid opportunities for sex, thereby diminishing the frequency of sex; or during sex, they avoid certain sexual activities that may trigger PTSS. Jessica purposely and effortfully stayed emotionally and sexually disengaged during sex to avoid triggers. Of course, this meant there was no sexual pleasure either. Avoidance or disengagement detracts from pleasure in the sexual experience.

Jessica felt damaged by the incest, a feeling that was reinforced by the gynecologist's subsequent abuse. "There is something fundamentally wrong with me," thought Jessica; "otherwise, my father would not have abused me, or I would have stopped it. My gynecologist could see it too; otherwise, he never would have abused me too." These thoughts made her burn with shame. Yet somehow, despite the flashbacks, the fear, the vigilance, the shame, and the negative self-talk that narrated her sexual encounters, Jessica never said no to sex with Justin. When he expressed concern, Jessica would reassure him that she just needed time, that she would be more comfortable with sex over time. But Jessica knew this was not true. Things were getting worse.

Childhood

Jessica had many of the risk factors for developing the sexual problems she was experiencing with Justin. These risk factors were evident in the story of her abuse, so it was important to understand the details of her history.

Jessica finally told her mother about the incest when the abuse escalated to oral sex and Jessica felt that she would surely choke to death if it continued. Her mother believed her but begged her not to tell anyone else, which meant that Jessica could not access therapy. Jessica's mother was not unsympathetic to her daughter, and the abuse stopped after the disclosure, but Jessica's mother was likely frightened. She depended on her husband's income, and she lived in a country where she had limited resources, no extended family, limited language skills, and ignorance about the legal system. Her husband worked long hours and a different shift from Jessica's mother, leaving little time for Jessica's parents to be together. Jessica's mother thought, erroneously, that this entirely explained the incest: "You have to understand, Jessica; your father is not himself. He is very sad and lonely. He made a mistake. He won't do this again. We must forgive and forget."

Jessica understood that she must not tell anyone or her father would have to go to jail, and that there would be great shame for the family, not to mention the dashed hopes of extended family members waiting in Korea for Jessica's parents to sponsor their immigration. So, with this heavy burden placed on her 10-year-old shoulders, Jessica kept the abuse to herself. She felt sorry for her parents and so could not be angry with them. She did not think it was possible for her to forgive, but she did her best to forget. In the isolation of her young mind, Jessica felt even more alienated from her American-born classmates and developed a deepening sense of shame.

In order to forget, Jessica tried not to show any outward signs of her damage, hoping this would counteract her sense of shame. Jessica became studious, perfectionistic, and highly anxious about her academic performance, which her teachers, falling prey to stereotypes, attributed to the pressures of coming from an Asian family. Jessica picked at her fingernails and made tiny cuts with a safety pin on her inner thighs and abdomen when she felt particularly bad and when she had intrusive memories of the abuse. She avoided interacting with her peers and did not date or socialize.

Jessica's high school classmates thought she was weird and aloof, and she was bullied (called names, laughed at, shoved aside in lines and hallways, and joked about). Even if she had wanted to, Jessica had virtually no options for romantic relationships as she was a social outcast. She discovered masturbation by accident when she was bathing and running water on her genitals. However, Jessica often thought about the abuse when she masturbated, and so after orgasm, she would take out a safety pin and scratch until she bled. Jessica suffered quietly, having nightmares, flashbacks, and most of all, hating herself. Then, at age 19, Jessica was sexually revictimized: She was abused by her gynecologist, who masturbated while pretending to conduct a medical exam.

It is with this history that Jessica presented for therapy. On the positive side, Jessica was smart; she had excelled academically and now held an MBA. She had a good job, and against all odds, she was engaged to a kind, caring, and supportive man.

The improbable story of Jessica's relationship started with a haircut for a job interview. Jessica became engaged to the man who cut and styled her hair, admittedly the first man she had ever let touch her. Their relationship started when Justin (the stylist) asked Jessica if she would help him set up his own salon business by assisting him with accounting and financial regulations. First, Jessica was Justin's client; then she was his accountant, his friend, his girlfriend, and his fiancée. Prior to having sex, Jessica told Justin about the sexual assault by the gynecologist, but not about the incest. She was too ashamed and also did not want Justin to hate her father or look down on her family. Justin knew that Jessica did not enjoy sex as much as he did; he attributed this to the abuse he knew about, her perfectionism, and her inexperience. He encouraged her to seek therapy.

Jessica's Therapy

Jessica told me from her initial phone call that she wanted to see me because she had been abused by the doctor in whose trial I had testified. We spent several sessions talking about the abuse she experienced with Dr. N, the gynecologist. Jessica went to Dr. N because of heavy bleeding during her last few menstrual cycles. She told her mother that the doctor seemed "weird," that he touched her vulva in a "creepy way," and that he appeared to be rubbing himself (his penis) with his hand. Her mother told her that the doctor likely saw many older women patients (Jessica's mother was Dr. N's patient as well) and that he should not be faulted for being excited when a young and attractive new patient came to him. (At trial, the defense attorney suggested that the doctor's behavior could also be explained by tight underwear or a case of "jock itch"—and I wish I was making that up, but I am not.) Jessica wondered why she had frozen during the gynecology exam, and she wondered why she could not just get over it. She was vague and made oblique references to her fear that her marriage would not work out. She did not mention incest. I looked for opportunities to talk with Jessica about various relational aspects that could be affected by her lack of trust in herself: communication, finances, friends, and as illustrated in the dialogue that follows, sex. The dotted lines below represent when the dialogue was not continuous.

JESSICA: I want to get married. I love Justin. He is an amazing guy, truly amazing. But how do I know that it's going to work?

ME: It will be hard to take a risk on marriage when you continue to doubt yourself; you can't know for sure that any relationship will work out. There's always risk.

. . . .

ME: Tell me about your sexual relationship with Justin. I'm asking because many women who have histories of sexual assault have difficulty enjoying sex. I'm wondering if that's true for you.

JESSICA: But really, was it *assault*? It was just once, and I never went back.

ME: Once counts. (*Jessica is quiet and looks down.*) Once counts. And once can hurt. So, it makes sense that sexual assault can hurt someone's sexuality going forward; it might not, but it's important to know.

JESSICA: It wasn't Dr. N who hurt me the most.

ME: Who hurt you the most?

Jessica went on to disclose the incest after checking with me that her reading of the mandated reporting laws was correct and that since she was an adult and there were no other children at risk, her disclosure could remain confidential. (She was correct. At the time I was seeing Jessica, this was the status of the mandated reporting law in New Jersey. Therapists should be aware of the current laws on mandated reporting applicable to the state or province in which they practice.) I asked Jessica, as I ask all my survivor patients, to tell me the story of the abuse. I tell them that it is important for two reasons: First, it will help us understand the connection to their present distress, and second, it will alleviate their sense of shame. I tell many of them, "Sexual abuse can only happen in secret, and keeping the secret has not helped you. Keeping it a secret makes it feel like it is your shame, not his. Talking about what you experienced makes it no longer a secret. The reason I want to know about what happened to you in the detail that we will talk about it is that shame can hide in the details."

When I say "shame can hide in the details," I mean that sometimes therapists make statements with good intentions, but patients may dismiss these statements if they feel the therapist does not have all the facts. For example, if a therapist says, "It's not your fault; you didn't do anything wrong," patients may think to themselves, "Well, but you don't know everything . . . you don't know that I asked to sleep in the bed with him . . . you don't know that it felt good to me at first . . . you don't know that he asked me if it was okay and I said yes." This is why I ask for details about the abuse.

Pulverman and Meston (2020) noted that, given the important and negative role that shame plays in the sexuality of survivors, treatments that target and reduce sexual shame are most likely to improve sexual outcomes. We naturally want to alleviate the distress that our patients suffer when they are processing difficult and painful subjects in therapy. Listening to stories of sexual abuse, and empathizing with the pain, fear, shame, and disgust that accompany disclosures, is extraordinarily difficult but necessary to alleviate the sense of shame.

The same guidelines apply to talking about the current sexuality of survivors as apply to talking about the past abuse: As you make the process of therapy transparent, you will make or propose connections between the past and the present difficulties, such that the reasons for asking certain questions are explicit. Survivors need to know why they are being asked to endure the sometimes painful process of therapy, and they need to know that they do not have to suffer. They can control the tempo of the therapeutic discussion.

ME: Jessica, we need to understand what exactly triggers the flashbacks. So I'm going to ask you questions about what is happening just before you have a flashback. I'm going to ask you about what you are doing, what Justin is doing, what you are thinking, feeling, or sensing at that moment. There may be more than one trigger, or not. It's possible that this part of therapy might itself trigger a flashback, or dissociation, or just get too difficult. If you feel any of those things might be happening, or if you just need a break, tell me, "Time for a break," or just raise your hand, and I'll stop so we can take a break. The most important thing is to go at the pace that's right for you.

. . . .

ME: Jessica, think back to the last time you had a flashback when you were having sex with Justin. (I want to orient her to a specific example, and I do this by asking about extraneous details: day of the week, time of day, what they were doing before, etc.)

. . . .

ME: (*summarizing what Jessica told me*) So, it was last Tuesday, and you were doing the dishes before you and Justin had sex. About 9 o'clock . . .

JESSICA: Yes, we ate late because of Justin's hours at the salon on Tuesday. It's his late night; otherwise, we cook and clean up together.

ME: Okay, so this night, because Justin had worked late, you were doing the dishes yourself. Then what happened?

JESSICA: Then we went to the bedroom and had sex.

ME: I know this sounds picky, but it may be important to know whether you were already thinking about having sex or if it was not yet on your mind.

JESSICA: Oh, ya. Like, was it a surprise? Not really; I'm pretty sure Justin would like sex every night. Well . . . I was a bit surprised because I thought he would be too tired. But he asked me if he should turn on the heat in the bedroom, which means, do I want to have sex with him.

ME: So when he said, "Do you want me to turn on the heat?" what happened?

JESSICA: I said yes, of course.

ME: You said yes. Did you feel yes?

JESSICA: If I'm being completely honest, I felt a bit like someone let the air out of my balloon. I was tired, and I wanted to go to sleep early.

ME: What made you decide to say yes instead of no?

This interchange about the initiation of sex provides helpful information (Does Jessica feel that she has agency in whether to have sex on a particular occasion?). It also sets the tone and cadence for subsequent questions about more sensitive aspects of her sexual experiences.

. . . .

ME: You remember feeling Justin's erection against your thigh. (*Jessica nods.*) What was going on in your head?

JESSICA: I'm thinking he is very happy and excited.

ME: And what are you feeling—emotionally?

JESSICA: I don't know if this is an emotion, but I feel cold. (*I nod.*) Well, okay, emotionally, I feel pressured. I'm feeling that I should be happy too, so maybe that's guilt; Justin would want me to be happy about this, but I feel cold.

ME: Cold.

JESSICA: (*anxiously*) And then I feel like I'm 10 years old, and I can smell the smell of my father's mouthwash, and I feel his breath, and I'm gagging. (*Jessica is crying.*)

ME: Let's stop here for a moment. Jessica, that makes a lot of sense. What you said makes a lot of sense. The feeling of Justin's erection makes you feel pressured to feel something you don't feel, to be happy for him and pleased about his erection.

JESSICA: I'm a terrible girlfriend; he deserves better. (*crying*)

ME: Jessica, that pressure you talked about; it sounds to me like the pressure you described feeling when your father was abusing you.

JESSICA: Oh, God, I know he wanted me to be happy. He really didn't want to hurt me. I don't believe that. So, I pretended to be happy about it. How could he know? He said, "Look what you did," and he laughed. And I laughed. And then he put his penis in my mouth. (*crying harder now and gagging*) Oh God, I think I'm going to be sick.

ME: (*placing the garbage pail in front of Jessica in case she does get sick; she doesn't*) Just breathe, Jessica. Take some deep breaths. You're here, in Princeton. In my office. Look around, Jessica. Look at the office, at the bookshelf, at the photograph of the elephants. (*Jessica is breathing regularly and looking around and wiping her eyes.*)

ME: Jessica, you don't have to feel anything about anyone's erection ever again if you don't want to. (*Jessica half laughs, half sobs.*) That was progress. That was hard, but that connection you just made was progress. Now we know that feeling pressure and feeling guilty triggers flashbacks.

JESSICA: I can't not have sex with Justin! I can't ask him not to have an erection. I can't tell him that I feel too much pressure.

ME: It's your choice whether or not to have sex with Justin, on a particular day, night, whenever. It's your choice. But you don't feel that it is a choice yet. So, we need to work on that. You can "not have sex with Justin." But I think not having sex with Justin ever is not the option you would choose.

Instead of leaving the session feeling depleted, scared, and hopeless, Jessica had some new insights, a feeling that she accomplished something, that she got somewhere today. (She often asked at the end of the session, "We got somewhere today, didn't we, doc?") Over time, Jessica began to tell herself, "I am choosing to have sex with Justin tonight." This meant, of course, that she did have to say no sometimes, to choose not to have sex with Justin on a particular occasion. She began to narrate their sexual encounters in her head, saying to herself, "I am choosing this. I am here with Justin. I love Justin. I don't have to be happy that he has an erection. I can feel what I want." When Jessica was no longer pressuring herself to feel happy for Justin, she began to use mindfulness and breathing exercises to slow racing thoughts and calm her anxiety. She learned to distinguish the rapid heartbeat of arousal from a panicked heart rate. Without the pressure to feel what she thought Justin wanted her to feel, Jessica could allow herself the opportunity to feel the sensuality (warmth, smooth, hard) and later the sexuality (arousal) of her sexual interactions with Justin. All these strategies helped Jessica stay present during sex with Justin and allowed her the opportunity to experience the pleasure of consensual sex.

Jessica did tell Justin about the incest. Midway through her therapy and well prior to their wedding date, Jessica told her parents that she was going to tell Justin, and then she told him. The incest was difficult for Justin to hear, especially since Jessica was asking him to have a relationship with her father. It helped that Justin had his own therapist to help him process this disclosure. "I don't want any more secrets," Jessica said. "Secrets make me feel bad about myself."

DANIEL'S STORY

For years Daniel tried to believe that his history of sexual abuse did not affect him. He primarily blamed his wife for his sexual unhappiness and thus justified his porn use and frequent visits to massage parlors offering happy endings. But high-profile stories in the media made the link between sexual abuse and sexual problems vividly real for Daniel. Interviews given by athletes, actors, and other famous men described childhood sexual abuse by trusted coaches, teachers, mentors, and parents. In these interviews, the men described the damage done to their ability to trust, to be intimate, and to be loving. Many of these men acknowledged multiple affairs, including having sex with sex workers. Daniel related to these stories. Aware that the clock was ticking and that he was aging out of the possibility of having a fulfilling sex life, Daniel came to therapy knowing he would have to talk about what happened to him decades earlier.

Childhood

Daniel was 2 years old when his father was killed in a car accident. After living happily with his grandparents, Daniel and his mother left that relatively peaceful home when his mother remarried. Daniel was 5 years old, and his stepfather turned out to be verbally and physically abusive to both Daniel and his mother. When Daniel was 12, his mother enrolled him in a youth group run by a local community organization. She wanted Daniel to have positive male role models and to have recreational and educational opportunities that she could not provide. His mother was pleased that Ken, the 37-year-old leader of the group, took a special interest in Daniel. The word was that Ken, a high school teacher, was a strict disciplinarian but a good man.

Daniel really liked the youth group, and a smaller group of five boys, Daniel among them, also went with Ken to baseball games, the movies, bowling, and other recreational activities that Daniel's family could ill afford. Soon Daniel was sleeping over at Ken's house on the weekends, first camping out on the living room sofa and, when the sofa was removed for reupholstering, sharing a king-sized bed with Ken. One night, Daniel awoke to find Ken touching his (Daniel's) penis. It appeared as though Ken was doing this in his sleep, so Daniel also pretended to be asleep. To his great embarrassment, however, Daniel ejaculated. He and Ken never spoke about the event.

On subsequent occasions when Daniel slept over at Ken's, Daniel tried to avoid a repeat occurrence by positioning his body away from Ken, clinging to the side of the bed, and trying to stay awake and vigilant until Ken fell asleep. But it did happen again. And again. Daniel felt trapped. He no longer knew what was real and what was not. In the mornings after sleeping over at Ken's, he could not remember what happened during the night. Daniel did not know it then, but he was likely dissociating. Trapped in Ken's bed, Daniel left his body.

Daniel knew that it alleviated the pressure on his mother to have him out of the house, and he also wanted to avoid being the object of his stepfather's wrath, but Daniel knew he could not keep staying with Ken, so he began hanging out with kids who stayed out late, crashed on each other's bedroom floors, did drugs, and engaged in petty crimes. His drug use corroborated his stepfather's negative opinion of Daniel, and the verbal abuse escalated.

Daniel's Therapy

When I met Daniel, it was more than 40 years after the abuse. He had never told anyone about it, except his wife. Before coming to see me, Daniel and his wife, Michelle, had gone to couples therapy at Daniel's insistence. Daniel wanted help navigating a better sex life with Michelle, who was a very reluctant participant in the process. However, when Michelle disclosed that Daniel had been sexually abused in childhood, their couples therapist insisted that first Daniel resolve the issues related to his abuse, and only then would they resume therapy for the sexual issues in their marriage.

Men who are abused as children often do not disclose, or delay their disclosure, meaning that many boys, and later men, never receive treatment for the impacts of their abuse. Some of the barriers to disclosure identified by male survivors include social norms (needing to appear strong and masculine and therefore unwilling to identify as a victim), internalized emotions such as shame and guilt, and interpersonal factors such as a mistrust of others and a fear of being labeled as gay (Easton et al., 2014).

All of the these factors were present in Daniel's case. Most disruptive, however, was the fear Daniel had of being labeled gay. It was this fear—either that he was gay (after all, he told me, he had an erection and ejaculated during the abuse), or that others would think he was gay (and then those men would insist on having sex with him)—that kept Daniel socially isolated. He never got close to other boys or men. In college, he was highly anxious about the possibility that his roommate was gay and that people he interacted with would assume he was gay. He avoided being with girls for fear of revealing his inexperience and being labeled a homosexual, so he did not date in high school or college. This homophobia puzzled Daniel because he did not consider himself to be "antigay"; he just did not want to be attracted to men. Nevertheless, his fear persisted, and this fear was not so much about prejudice but about the deep fear that the sexual abuse had damaged him and that, as a result, Daniel would never enjoy sex with a woman.

I did not agree with the couples therapist's decision to stop treatment with Daniel and Michelle, but that was not my call to make. To Daniel, it was an abrupt, unwarranted, and unwanted termination. He felt blamed for the sexual problems in his marriage, and he assumed the therapist saw him as damaged, something he saw every time he looked in the mirror, but something he sought desperately to hide from the outside world. According to Daniel, Michelle now felt vindicated in her belief that there was nothing she needed to change, only that Daniel needed to deal with his abuse in order to be happy with their sexual relationship as is.

Daniel was more desperate for help than his wife understood. Time was running out; he was aging, and he despaired of ever enjoying sex with a woman. Unbeknownst to Michelle, Daniel was a regular at the massage parlor where "happy endings" could be purchased for a healthy tip. Daniel also masturbated frequently to porn featuring actresses portraying college students (for example, a favorite theme was sex on spring break), and he was highly anxious that he would be sexually inappropriate with the young women he interacted with at work.

Daniel would fit into the category of being both sexually inhibited (having no desire for sex with his wife) and sexually disinhibited (going to massage parlors, frequently using porn, and constantly fantasizing about other women). Daniel was clear that he did not enjoy having sex with his wife, although they had sex on a weekly or biweekly basis. Daniel said that he had to fantasize about other women in order to get and maintain an erection with his wife. He had difficulty reaching orgasm, even using fantasy, when he was with her. Sex often ended only after Daniel had vigorously masturbated to orgasm. Daniel felt that his orgasm was a requirement and that Michelle would be hurt if he did not experience an orgasm with her.

Daniel loved his wife and his family (they had three daughters) and his life in general. His upper-middle-class lifestyle far exceeded his dreams when he was a young boy. But Daniel hated having, yet again, a secret. He did not want the stress of leading a dual life, and he desperately wanted to put it all together, but he could not. He could not imagine having good sex with his wife, and he could not imagine partnering with any of the women in his fantasies or with the sex workers at the massage parlors.

DANIEL: I just can't enjoy sex with my wife.

ME: I know it distresses you that you don't enjoy having sex with Michelle.

DANIEL: I know, I know, we've been through this before. I know you think that if I just ask for what I want, everything will be fine. But I can't do it.

ME: Well, I don't think everything will be fine, but it might be one step toward enjoying sex with Michelle, at least a little bit.

DANIEL: She's not interested. If she were—she would do those things already. And if I ask her, then I'll have to like it, won't I? . . . Anyway, she won't do it right.

ME: So, if you ask for something, you're afraid you won't enjoy it anyway?

DANIEL: Yes, and then it will be worse.

ME: Daniel, you don't have to feel anything that you don't feel. You don't have to enjoy sex that you don't like. But you focus on doing it, not experiencing it. You keep doing it, despite the fact that you don't enjoy it.

DANIEL: I enjoy the massage.

ME: Yes. But you're not supposed to, so you don't pressure yourself.

DANIEL: I know, I've thought about that: that I like sex that's wrong.

Our conversation continues as we explore the possibility that Daniel is turned on by sex he should not be having. And that may be right, but I want to understand the mechanisms at play that would allow Daniel to enjoy sex under certain circumstances and not others. Daniel's fantasy, if you will, is that the women giving him the massage are happy to see him because he is physically fit and is a nice person who treats them well, unlike the other customers he imagines they have. The massage allows him to relax, and he knows that he will tip them well, whether he gets aroused or not. Exploring the conditions under which Daniel can enjoy sex, which will allow us to understand the mechanisms by which he does and does not get turned on, requires talking explicitly about sex. Here is a brief excerpt from a session with Daniel:

ME: So you're on the massage table. What's happening in your body?

DANIEL: I'm kind of spaced out, to be clear. But she's touching me all over, not on my junk, to be clear. But near it. Teasing, you know?

ME: Do you have an erection?

DANIEL: I do. Not all the time, but most of the time.

ME: Okay, but you're spaced out? Do you feel turned on?

DANIEL: Ya, I'm hard. I don't know, I'm just feeling really good.

ME: What about when you ejaculate?

DANIEL: Oh, I don't.

ME: You don't ejaculate? I thought that's what a happy ending was.

DANIEL: I get really hard. Then she says, "Take that home to your wife."

ME: Oh, this is interesting—do you ever ejaculate when you get a massage?

DANIEL: No, never have. I usually go home and jerk off.

ME: Why don't you "take the erection home to your wife"?

DANIEL: (*laughing*) It wouldn't last that long! It's about a half-hour drive, and I go get a massage when Michelle is out of the house. But I don't think I would anyway. I'd be too guilty.

When Daniel told me he got massages with happy endings, I assumed that meant he ejaculated, because that is usually what "happy endings" means. This example highlights the importance of not making assumptions about what patients mean when they are talking about sex, especially when they use a catchphrase or colloquial expression. Now, several months later, I know that Daniel never ejaculated at the massage parlor but always did (he felt he had to) with Michelle. Daniel and I spent time in therapy processing his feelings about his unwanted ejaculations during the sexual abuse. Daniel got in touch with the anger he felt at his body for betraying him by ejaculating when he did not want to. Despite the information I was happy to supply about the ease with which teenage boys ejaculate, Daniel allowed himself no excuse. The only time he felt relaxed during sex was with sex workers; otherwise, he pressured himself to have an orgasm with Michelle and worried about being gay.

I asked Daniel why he was unable to ejaculate during intercourse. Daniel replied, "I don't know, I get lost; sometimes I'm worrying that I'm not going to cum because I'm gay, but sometimes I just space out until Michelle tells me to snap out of it. By then, I'm losing my erection, so I have to masturbate to cum." Shame, dissociation during sex with Michelle, and the traumatic sexualization of the past are all at least partially responsible for his lack of pleasure with his wife. As many of the theories suggest, it seemed to be everything, all at once, that was affecting Daniel's sexuality. His coping strategies of enjoying pornography and hiring sex workers further alienated him from the potential for pleasurable sex with Michelle.

Daniel's original goal for therapy was to be able to enjoy sex with his wife, even though he immediately dismissed this as impossible to achieve. We agreed to a revised goal of trying to stay present during sex and to focus more on his own body and his own desires. Slowly, over the course of a couple of years of therapy, Daniel connected with his body, only to become aware of the transactional nature of the massage parlor sex and how disconnected he actually felt there. Connecting to his body during sexual activity and becoming aware of his arousal calmed his panic about being gay.

Sex with Michelle continued to be routine and effortful. But as the fantasy of massage sex receded, Daniel began showing real interest in trying to enjoy sex with Michelle. He still did not want to ask her for anything sexual, and he continued to express pessimism: "I would like to enjoy sex with my wife, but I don't think it's really possible." Instead of focusing on pleasure, I suggested to Daniel that we work on just being more connected—with himself and with Michelle—during sex. There was no pressure to feel anything.

One big accomplishment was having Daniel connect with Michelle when he had an orgasm. Daniel fantasized about other women to become sufficiently aroused to ejaculate. This kept him disconnected from Michelle leading up to, during, and after his orgasm (as he felt guilty). So, I suggested that when Daniel reached the point of ejaculatory inevitability (a physiological point at which ejaculation is inevitable; see Appendix B), he could open his eyes just before he ejaculated to see Michelle. I thought it might intimately connect them, but it had a different, albeit positive, outcome. Daniel saw Michelle and noticed that she was pleased he had ejaculated, but he could also tell that she was just relieved that sex could be over. The idea that he needed to ejaculate for her because she wanted that (the way Ken wanted it) was rather suddenly dispelled. The emotional connection he sought came after he ejaculated, allowing him to enjoy cuddling with Michelle.

Daniel is continuing his work of surviving. Sex is less effortful with Michelle, but not magically erotic. Daniel still goes to the massage parlor, but not as often, and he feels less of a need to go there. I also encouraged Daniel to socialize with men, thereby adding an element of exposure therapy to his obsessive fears. His panic about being gay has diminished to the extent that he has joined a running group with other men to train for a half marathon. He still does not shower at the gym with them, but he is okay with that. It was emotionally difficult for me, at first, to listen to Daniel talk about his fears of being gay. I very much wanted to dispel his belief that being gay was bad. I knew, however, that if I did this, I ran the risk of further shaming him. I also knew two other things: It was my discomfort I was looking to alleviate, not his, and the way he articulated his fears reflected an adolescent boy's panic, so educating the adult man he was now about same-sex attractions would not have been helpful.

WHY MUST I SUFFER FOR WHAT SOMEONE ELSE DID? A NOTE ABOUT WORKING WITH PARTNERS OF SURVIVORS

Jessica's fiancé, Justin, was already in individual therapy when Jessica moved in with him. His own therapy helped Justin deal with the emotional difficulties he encountered when Jessica had flashbacks, or when she would not tell him what she wanted. It was very helpful for him to be in therapy when he learned of the incest, and he had to work through his own feelings about the fact that Jessica had not told him about it earlier.

Daniel's wife, Michelle, also went to therapy. Despite what Daniel chose to think, she did care, and she did notice that he did not enjoy sex. She just did not know what to do about it. She was an anxious person who was always trying to do the right thing, but she did not know what the right thing was when it came to sex. She assumed that Daniel was not attracted to her anymore, and she was highly anxious that he would leave her. She shared these insights from her own therapy with Daniel, and this saddened him and helped him resolve to continue to work on things in therapy.

Our work with partners of survivors aims to help them focus on their own issues as they cope with the challenges of being intimately involved with someone who has a history of abuse. Some partners want to become the therapist for the person they love, putting their own needs aside to help. Others become angry and mistakenly assume that they are being punished unfairly; in turn, they may make unfair demands on their partner. As survivors work in their own therapy to focus on their mental, emotional, and sexual well-being, partners are well served when they do the same.

Working with survivors and their partners in couples therapy will require many of the same skills and sensitivities addressed in this chapter. This includes being transparent about the process of therapy and focusing on staying present in their bodies and relationships.

SUMMARY

There is a strong connection between sexual abuse suffered in childhood and sexual problems experienced in adulthood. While several pathways have been explored, research points to the additive effect of many risk factors. Depending on the unique elements in the patient's history and current presentation, therapy may focus on alleviating shame, building trust, tolerating anxiety, and developing intimate attachments.

This chapter focused on childhood sexual abuse, but many of the factors responsible for adult sexual difficulties are present in other (nonsexual) forms of childhood abuse, neglect, and maltreatment. Nonsexual traumatic experiences in childhood also negatively affect adult sexuality, and the same treatment strategies outlined in this chapter will apply to therapy with survivors of nonsexual forms of abuse.

Survivor patients would love to be restored to the idealized version of who they could have been if the abuse had never occurred. But working with survivors requires that we focus on the present and the future as they seek to enjoy sex. Some of the sensitivities and skills required for this work are part of the skill set of most therapists, including empathy, listening with compassion, and helping patients regulate their emotions and stay present in the moment. But a very important component of the work with survivors who want to improve their enjoyment of sex is talking about sex explicitly: what happened in the past and what is happening in the present. Shame hides in the details, and the path forward is often found in those details as well.

It is painful for therapists to watch patients revisit traumatic events, but working with survivors is incredibly gratifying. Often for the first time, survivors are not in this alone; there is someone else who understands and knows what happened to them in detail. And there is someone who recognizes the vital importance of their desire to reclaim their sexuality from their abusive past.

7 KINKY SEX

Even with years of experience, I can still feel a bit overwhelmed, intimidated, or somehow just not up to the task of working with a patient who has a sexual problem I have never before encountered. So please know that there are times I have had to take my own advice: to trust the skills I have as a psychotherapist to see me through. This is especially relevant in the context of kinky sex, which is the focus of this chapter. For example, I could not have known that one day I would encounter a young man with a sneeze fetish.

JEREMY'S STORY

Jeremy was 17 and entering college, full of social anxiety after having been schooled virtually during the global COVID-19 pandemic. In the first months of therapy, I listened as Jeremy told me about his anxieties, as together we discussed ways he could navigate life in the dorm after almost 2 years of socially isolated living. We created hierarchies of socially difficult situations, role-played scenarios, and practiced breathing and relaxation exercises so that Jeremy could work his way through the feared interactions. Relating to

https://doi.org/10.1037/0000483-008
Talking About Sex in Psychotherapy: A Guide for Every Therapist, by K. S. K. Hall

his female peers outside of the classroom was at the top of the list in terms of fears and difficulties, and when we began to talk about sex, Jeremy told me about his sneeze fetish.

Truth be told, a sneeze fetish was outside my comfort zone. Even before the global pandemic that would make most of us cringe at the sound or sight of a sneeze, I really did not like people sneezing around me or near me. And so the fact that someone could not only find sneezing arousing but also believe he could be aroused and have an orgasm only when there was a sneeze was incomprehensible to me. In my initial panic, I thought, "I need to find a sneeze fetish expert and refer Jeremy to that person." Of course, there is no such person.

I had to remember that Jeremy was like many other college freshmen, eager and anxious about the social and sexual opportunities that awaited him. He wanted to meet people, make friends, be liked, and have sex, but he felt there was something wrong with him, something that would render him socially and sexually unappealing. Again, this is not an unusual clinical presentation for a person with anxiety and low self-esteem—except, in Jeremy's case, the thing that he thought was wrong with him was arousal to sneezing.

FETISHES, PARAPHILIAS, AND KINKS

A *fetish* is defined as the experience of intense sexual arousal from an inanimate object or a body part that is not usually considered to be sexual (American Psychiatric Association, 2013). Jeremy was intensely aroused by a sneezing nose. He had diagnosed himself with a sneeze fetish before even entering treatment. I was not about to argue with him; after all, he was right. A fetish is considered a *paraphilia*, which, as you may recall from Chapter 1, is "sexual interest other than interest in genital stimulation or preparatory fondling with phenotypically normal, physically mature, consenting human partners" (American Psychiatric Association, 2022, p. 779).

The term paraphilia, like its *Diagnostic and Statistical Manual of Mental Disorders* (*DSM*; American Psychiatric Association, 2022) definition, is a bit of a mouthful. It also carries negative connotations. For this reason, many people prefer to use the broader and more positive term *kink*, which encompasses a wider range of unusual sexual interests, such as fetishes; exhibitionism; and bondage and discipline, dominance and submission, and sadism and masochism (BDSM). Ortmann (2020) stated, "Kink is an umbrella term for the less-traveled path of human sexual adventures. The word *kink*, like the word *bent*, indicates a turning away from the mainstream, a twist on what is considered 'normal'" (p. 297). Ortmann (2020) also notes that kink can be used to describe an identity or orientation, as many feel that "their kinkiness is an inherent part of their sexuality and therefore an important part of their overall identity" (p. 297). When patients refer to themselves as "kinky," I am happy to use their terminology. For the purposes of this chapter, however, I refer to people who are on the less-traveled path of human sexual adventures as *sexual minorities* (even though there will be times when this is statistically doubtful). In this chapter, sexual minorities does not necessarily mean lesbian, gay, bisexual, and transgender (LGBT), although sexual minorities can be LGBT. And when summarizing the research literature, I will be using the terms used in the original research papers, which is mostly paraphilias.

THE DEVELOPMENT OF KINKY SEXUAL INTERESTS

It is tempting to speculate that Jeremy developed his fetish as a coping mechanism in response to trauma—for example, to help him gain some sense of mastery over a frightening symptom of a new and deadly disease epidemic. However, Jeremy reported that he had happened upon sneeze porn (Who knew there was such a thing?) years earlier when he was in middle school, and he found it incredibly arousing. His hopes to have some sexual experiences in high school did not materialize because of the COVID-19 lockdown. With his lack of experience (except for sneeze porn), Jeremy found himself highly anxious about sex. He did not know why he was so aroused by seeing a woman sneeze; he just was.

The short answer to the question of the etiology of atypical, paraphilic, or kinky sexual interests is that we do not know how or why people develop the sexual preferences they do. There are several hypotheses, each with limited empirical evidence: that paraphilias are a result of learned experiences (classical or operant conditioning); that they represent ways of coping with anxiety or other psychological disorders; or that they are a result of trauma (Fox et al., 2022). The fact is, however, that when we are talking about kink, or paraphilias, we are referencing not a singular entity but rather an array of sexual preferences (e.g., interest in dominance, voyeurism, fetishes for body parts, fetishes for inanimate objects, masochism, exhibitionism). Perhaps the only thing that connects these disparate interests is the assumption that they are not "normal." Many of the theories of etiology rely on the understanding that the sexual interests that have been defined as paraphilic are indeed statistically unusual, an assumption that may not currently be correct.

So perhaps a better question is "What makes a person kinky?" Why do some people enjoy the less-traveled path of human sexual adventures while others stick to the main road? Maybe kinky people are simply more adventurous; after all, kinky people often have high levels of sexual interest in a broad range of sexual activities (Joyal, 2021). It is likely that there are multiple routes to developing sexual interests and preferences (kinky or mainstream), including biological, psychological, social, and environmental factors. In other words, we are back to the basic building blocks of all forms of human sexuality as described by the biopsychosocial model.

JEREMY'S THERAPY

My working hypothesis was that Jeremy had developed an arousal to sneezes because he happened upon sneeze porn at a particular point in his sexual development when he was easily aroused and when his sexual arousal was highly malleable (around puberty for Jeremy). Jeremy's social and sexual anxiety (fueled in part by his social isolation) led him to continue to focus on sneezing as a source of sexual pleasure, rather than on the person he might one day be with, as this possibility made him anxious. The more Jeremy relied on sneeze porn for sexual satisfaction, the more socially anxious he became because he felt, in his words, "like a freak."

I confess that I was perplexed by Jeremy's fetish. I kept wondering why. What is so erotic about sneezing? But I was asking the wrong question. I did not need to understand why Jeremy was excited by a forceful expulsion of air through the nose and mouth. What I needed to understand was why Jeremy was not aroused by much else. This was a bit of an "aha!" moment for me. Most of my patients with extreme anxiety have a similarly rigid pattern of sexual responding, even though many of them engage in mainstream sexual activities. They find a pattern or a routine that works for them sexually, and they stick with it; the sequence of events that comprise the act of sex is relentlessly and rigidly fixed.

When working with these patients, I help them expand their repertoire of sexual activities while helping them to process and reduce their anxiety so that they are open to becoming aroused by new or different sources of pleasure. Expanding what Jeremy found arousing, beyond sneezing, became the goal by expanding the source of his arousal to include the person who was sneezing. It was what Jeremy wanted as well: to have a relationship and to be sexual within that relationship. So, we created yet another hierarchy, with sneezing at the base (the surefire way to be aroused and experience orgasm); the idea of a sneeze coming on; the fantasy of a sneeze; a nose, eyes, a face; and finally the whole person completing and topping the list as the most difficult situation for Jeremy's arousal and orgasm.

At this point in the therapy, Jeremy was in college and struggling socially. His therapy homework was to begin masturbation in his usual fashion, by fantasizing about a woman sneezing, and then to expand the picture in his mind of the nose, the face, and the whole person who was sneezing. At the point of orgasm, Jeremy was to try to imagine a whole person, or at least a whole face. Over time, Jeremy was able to become aroused by fantasies or pornography that included not overt sneezing but only the imagined possibility of the woman sneezing. When Jeremy felt it was possible that he could be attracted to a woman who had a nose that could one day sneeze, he began to put himself in social situations. As he became more adept socially, and less anxious, he began to consider whether he was attracted to a female peer based on imagining her sneeze.

Toward the end of his freshman year, Jeremy began seeing a female classmate who, among her other qualities, had a rather pronounced nose. His first orgasm with a partner happened during intercourse, where he focused on her nose and imagined that nose sneezing. We worked together to make sure that Jeremy was not reducing his partner to a nose but also taking in the rest of her and attending to her needs and desires during sex. The girl with the large nose broke up with Jeremy, as often happens in college romances. Jeremy took it well. Over the summer, he had another successful sexual and emotional relationship with a female peer, and he felt confident entering sophomore year that he could navigate sexually and socially. Make no mistake: Jeremy was still aroused by sneeze porn and sneezing, and he greatly enjoyed allergy season. But his enjoyment of sex now encompassed much more; his sexual interests extended to actual and potential partners.

This outcome for Jeremy reflects what most kinky people experience; most are also interested in and engage in traditional sexual behaviors as well as their kink practices. Fetishes, like most sexual preferences, deny overt efforts to extinguish them (Krause, 2023). Jeremy's anxiety kept him from enjoying other sources of sexual pleasure. Therapy reduced that anxiety and allowed him to enjoy the partnered sex he so wanted, along with the sneeze fetish that continued to arouse him.

THE PREVALENCE OF PARAPHILIAS (HOW COMMON IS KINK?)

A surprisingly high number of people acknowledge arousal to sexual behaviors and activities that are not mainstream. In large-scale population-based surveys, a significant number of men and women (a third to almost half of the samples) report paraphilic sexual interest, sexual behavior, and sexual arousal and fantasies, as well as viewing pornography depicting paraphilic activity. In these surveys, the number of men reporting paraphilic interests is higher, often three times higher than the number of women (Bártová et al.,

2021; Joyal et al., 2015; Joyal & Carpentier, 2017). While more people are interested in and aroused by paraphilic behaviors than have engaged in them, a significant percentage of people acknowledge that they have engaged in at least some of these activities (one quarter to one third of the samples). In other words, many people are aroused by, or engage in, what are often considered to be atypical, kinky, or paraphilic sexual activities.

The most commonly reported paraphilic interests and behaviors are voyeurism, fetishism, frotteurism, and masochism. In the survey conducted by Joyal and Carpentier (2017), voyeurism was assessed by the following question: "Have you ever been sexually aroused while watching a stranger, who was unaware of your presence, while they were nude, were undressing, or were having sexual relations?" Fetishism was assessed by this question: "Have you ever been sexually aroused by an inanimate nonsexual object? Please note that a vibrator does not enter into this category." Frotteurism was assessed thus: "Have you ever been sexually aroused by touching or by rubbing yourself against a stranger?" The question about masochism was this: "Have you ever been sexually aroused while suffering, being dominated, or being humiliated?"

BDSM is an initialism for bondage, discipline, dominance, submission, sadism, and masochism, a collection of power-based sexual interests and behaviors (Ortmann, 2020). Interest and engagement in power-based sexual activities are high in the general population, with one survey finding that almost 70% of men and women are interested in this type of activity (Holvoet et al., 2017). Specific activities may include the use of restraints, impact play such as spanking and slapping, submissive kneeling, and using blindfolds (Herbenick et al., 2017). In the BDSM community, the erotic potential of power may also be reflected in relationship constellations based on dominance and submissiveness. Describing these relationships is beyond the scope of this chapter, however, and the interested reader is referred to Ortmann (2020) and to the resources listed in Appendix D.

PARAPHILIAS AND PSYCHOPATHOLOGY

So if the paraphilias represent sexual interests that are really not that atypical, what is it that makes people and professionals still think of them as deviant? One often-cited reason is that there is a correlation between paraphilias and psychopathology. The truth is that the strong association that was assumed to exist between psychopathology and paraphilias was based on early studies that recruited participants from correctional facilities, as well as from forensic and psychiatric settings, so there was a high probability of confounding variables. At present, there is no strong evidence supporting the view that an interest in a wide range of sexual activities and consensually engaging in diverse sexual behaviors are symptomatic of underlying psychopathology. The exception to this conclusion involves those sexual interests that are indeed rare in the general population: engaging in sexual activities with prepubertal children, animals, corpses, and excrement. These activities may be indicative of underlying psychopathology, but this speculation awaits empirical validation (Joyal, 2021).

Note that there is an important difference between a paraphilia and a diagnosis of paraphilic disorder. In response to the overwhelming evidence that most paraphilias are not, in and of themselves, pathological, the *DSM-5* clarified that paraphilias should be the focus of treatment only if they cause personal distress or impairment, or involve coercion and harm to others (American Psychiatric Association, 2013). So, a paraphilic disorder is diagnosed only if the paraphilic interest causes distress or impairment in an important area of life (previously, having a paraphilic sexual interest was enough to warrant a diagnosis). A paraphilic disorder is also diagnosed when paraphilic interests (including, and especially, sexual sadism and pedophilia) are acted upon with partners who either do not or cannot consent. Note that engaging in any sexual behavior with a nonconsenting partner is criminal.

It is likely that social values have had an undue influence over what sexual interests are considered deviant or pathological (Moser & Kleinplatz, 2020). Consider the fact that in the late 1800s, oral sex, or more precisely cunnilingus, was thought to be a sign of pathological masochism (Krafft-Ebing, 1892). Currently, oral sex is not only a popular sexual fantasy but also a frequently engaged-in sexual behavior (Joyal & Carpentier, 2017). The popularity of BDSM is another case in point. Women's interest in BDSM used to be considered a symptom of sexual trauma. Recent studies have failed to find that this is true. Rather, it appears that women's arousal to BDSM (in fantasy or in activity) is indicative of a high interest in and enjoyment of sex (Ortmann, 2020). Christian Joyal (2021), a professor at the University of Quebec at Trois-Rivières in Canada and a specialist in cognitive neuropsychology and forensic neuroscience, has reviewed the literature and has an even stronger assertion: "Studies strongly suggest that the psychological health of BDSM practitioners is similar to (if not better than) that of non-practitioners" (p. 98).

It is a step in the right direction that, in order to diagnose a paraphilic disorder, there must now be distress or impairment. But diagnosing a paraphilic disorder solely on the basis of distress or impairment is still inherently problematic. Distress and impairment often result from the negative attitudes and discriminatory behavior that sexual minorities often experience or fear. While it is certainly a valid focus of treatment to help people troubled by their sexual preferences (as I did with Jeremy), the diagnosis of paraphilic disorder puts undue emphasis on the unusual sexual interest rather than the difficulties inherent in coping with negative reactions and discrimination. Therapists often help people who struggle because they do not live up to personal, familial, societal, or cultural expectations and who have internalized this negativity. And we do this without pathologizing the person, their values, their behavior, or their culture. So we can also do this without pathologizing their sexual preferences. In other words, psychotherapists have the skills to work with sexual minority (kinky) patients.

In my experience, people rarely come to therapy wishing to rid themselves of an erotic fantasy or enjoyable behavior unless they are experiencing or anticipating relational difficulties. What often brings people to therapy is the distress they feel about either needing to hide or wishing to incorporate their sexual interests into a relationship. The following case describes the treatment of a man who had a strong interest in BDSM and who found himself unable to make changes to his behavior despite the jeopardy it presented to his marriage.

AHMAD'S STORY

Ahmad was a very successful man and the pride of his family and community. A first-generation Palestinian Muslim, he had risen from near poverty to establish his own successful law practice specializing in medical malpractice. Early in his career, he won a precedent-setting case that allowed him to open his own law firm and hire several associates. He was featured in newspapers and law journals. He was a sought-after speaker at law conferences. He was a good lawyer. He was a good Muslim, he was a good son, he was a good father, and he was a good husband. Ahmad was a good man. And he was a tortured man.

Ahmad came to therapy in a panic. His wife found leather BDSM gear, including a harness and collar, in a suitcase that was stored in his home office. Ahmad explained to his upset wife that they were evidence for an upcoming trial. This was a lie. He hoped his wife believed him, but he knew she was suspicious—and newly vigilant. This was a close call, and Ahmad was panicked. "Help me. Help me stop going to leather bars. Please. This could ruin me." The term *leather* is often used as shorthand for BDSM, especially in gay male BDSM communities, because of community members' propensity to wear leather. In Ahmad's case, *leather bars* referred to those bars frequented by the gay male BDSM community.

In his early 40s, Ahmad looked more like a man in his mid-twenties. He was tall, slender, and muscular, with olive skin, jet-black hair, and deep brown eyes framed by large lashes. He was, by all measures, an extremely handsome man. In our very first session, after the preliminaries, this encounter occurred:

AHMAD: I'm bisexual.

ME: (*nodding*) Okay.

AHMAD: No, it's important. It's important that you believe me.

ME: Why would I not believe you?

AHMAD: I've been in therapy before, and I'm tired of being told that I'm really gay. I'm tired of being told that I need to come to terms with that and embrace it. So, I need to know—do you believe that there is such a thing as bisexuality?

ME: I do. In fact, I'm quite certain there is such a thing as bisexuality.

AHMAD: (*audibly sighing*) Well, that's good. I'm glad that's settled.

Bisexuality is an often-misunderstood sexual orientation. Ahmad had been told that his bisexuality was evidence of an unstable attachment style, ambivalence about his own masculinity due to the trauma of his father's abandonment, a symptom of narcissistic personality disorder, or, in reality, internalized homophobia—a mask for his unacceptable attraction to men. Previous therapists had filtered sexual information that was unfamiliar and confusing to them through a lens that made intuitive sense to them—in this case, through a psychotherapeutic lens of pathology. Ahmad wanted help managing his sexual behavior. To presume that his sexual orientation was the root cause of his problems would be alienating as well as unhelpful and incorrect. To deny Ahmad the right to define his sexual orientation would also be countertherapeutic; in other words, past therapists were mistaken when they blamed Ahmad's bisexuality for his problems and when they tried to tell Ahmad that he was not bisexual.

Sexual orientation typically refers to an enduring pattern of sexual and romantic attraction, historically centered on gender: attraction to men, women, or both genders. Sexual orientations other than heterosexuality are not pathological or deviant. The American Psychological Association (2022) has clearly stated that "same-sex sexual and romantic attractions, feelings, and behaviors are normal and positive variations of human sexuality" (para. 19) and that psychologists should refrain from engaging in therapeutic endeavors to change sexual orientation given the lack of evidence that these interventions are helpful and the evidence that they are often, in fact, harmful.

Ahmad and other patients should be believed when they identify as gay, heterosexual, or bisexual. However, it should be noted that these three distinct sexual orientations do not make sense to everyone. Many sexual minority individuals do not find the heterosexual–homosexual continuum relevant to their experiences. Instead, they talk about being attracted to personality rather than gender, being attracted to different genders in different ways, and being attracted to gender nonconforming individuals (Weitzman, 2007). Labels, if they are used, include terms such as *pansexual, open, unsure, bicurious,* and *gender blind* (Manley et al., 2015), as well as *queer* and *questioning*. Whatever the label, or if your patient eschews labels, the important point remains to listen without judgment to your patient's experience. But let us return to Ahmad, who wanted help with his sexual behavior, not with his sexual orientation. "Help me. Stop me from going to leather bars. Please. This could ruin me."

History

Ahmad was born in Chicago to immigrant parents from Palestine. When he was 10 years old, his father left the family and relocated to Arizona, where he started a new family with an American woman of European descent. Ahmad has had no contact with him since. After his father left, and for reasons still unclear to him, Ahmad was sent to live with his maternal grandparents in Palestine. His two younger brothers continued to live with their mother. Ahmad knew that Palestine was not the safest place to raise children ("So why did my mother send me there?"), but even with the undertones of danger, Ahmad thought his grandmother was stricter and more vigilant than necessary and stricter in comparison to the restrictions placed on his friends. Ahmad was allowed only to go to school and to play in his grandparents' small yard but not to go to friends' homes, cafés, or parks. He was lonely and became studious because he lacked other diversions. His grandfather took him to pray at the mosque most mornings and evenings, which Ahmad grew to appreciate.

At age 16, he returned to the United States to finish high school and attend university. He continued to be studious and withdrawn once back in the United States, and he continued to pray at the mosque. In law school he lived in New York, away from family for the first time; he no longer went to a mosque for prayer, and he began to have sex with men. His first sexual experience was vividly recalled by Ahmad. He was on the subway and noticed that the attractive man sitting opposite him was staring. Somehow, he knew that a sexual invitation was being extended, and without words being exchanged, he followed the man out of the subway car and into a leather bar.

Throughout law school, Ahmad had sex exclusively (and secretly) with men. Ahmad believed he was heterosexual and attributed the sex he had with men as opportunistic; his faith prohibited sex with women before marriage. By his own choice, he never had an emotional or social relationship with his male sexual partners. Meanwhile, as graduation approached, his mother suggested to Ahmad that he think about marriage. Ahmad deferred, saying he preferred to wait until he had his first job at a law firm. Ahmad continued to have sex with men, primarily in leather bars. The second of two women his mother introduced him to became Ahmad's wife once he was settled in his law practice. He described his wife, Layla, as beautiful and kind, and his only complaint was that she was overly anxious with their children. He described their sex life as enjoyable and emotionally fulfilling, but there was none of that first-time amazement he experienced at the leather bar. He and his wife were both shy and nervous on their wedding night.

Ahmad stopped going to leather bars once he was married, intending to be faithful to his wife and understanding that the rationale of being able to have sex with men only prior to marriage no longer held true. Sex became less frequent and less pleasurable after the children were born, and Ahmad began going to leather bars again, at first sporadically and then about once a week. It was at this time that Ahmad admitted to himself that he was bisexual. While Ahmad felt that an occasional visit to the leather bar was a reasonable accommodation to his bisexual orientation, his almost weekly visits were too much for his comfort. When Ahmad came to therapy, he was full of fear: fear that his marriage and his reputation would be destroyed if his sexual behavior was discovered. He felt unable to keep everything together. He felt he was about to fall apart.

"Help me. Help me stop going to leather bars. Please. This could ruin me."

Using a Cultural Framework

It is often difficult for therapists to work effectively with patients who have sexual practices and interests that they do not understand. The risk is that therapists will mistake their personal discomfort for their professional judgment. It is important to remember, as I did with Jeremy, that the struggles of our sexual minority patients are not that different from the struggles of many of our patients. It can also be very helpful to refer to the literature on working with cultural minorities, another area in which we must try to distinguish our biases from our clinical judgment. In fact, the American Psychological Association (2022) has suggested that multiculturally competent treatment models may provide a useful foundation for work with sexual minorities, especially for sexual minority patients like Ahmad, who are also members of underrepresented ethnic, religious, racial, and cultural groups.

The stress placed on ethnic and sexual minority patients is tremendous. While many ethnic minorities depend on their families and communities for support, some of these supports are withdrawn for sexual minority persons (Nichols, 2013). Ahmad's success was built upon his mother's hard work, his grandparents' care, his faith community's support, and financial help from friends and family. He could not and would not jeopardize their support, and he wanted to remain a responsible member of his community.

Hall and Graham (2012, 2014, 2020) proposed a model of culturally sensitive sex therapy that requires exquisite listening: listening without judgment to the sexual and relational narratives of patients. This approach is similar to other models of cross-cultural psychotherapy, most specifically the cultural humility approach (Hook et al., 2016). Both of these approaches stress the need for therapists to learn from patients those things that the therapist does not understand regarding the patients' cultures and, as Hall and Graham emphasize, their sexuality. I started by listening to Ahmad. It was an important distinction to understand that I could ask Ahmad about his bisexuality without questioning or pathologizing his sexual orientation. I asked because I was interested in him.

ME: Ahmad, tell me about your experience of being bisexual.

AHMAD: Well, I really didn't come to terms with it until fairly recently. I kind of thought straight men have sex with men when they can't have sex with women. That's what I did, what I still do, I guess. I mean, I didn't have any sex with men when I was first married. But when we had kids, then I started to go back out.

ME: Back out to leather bars? (*Ahmad nods yes.*) Okay, so for a long time you assumed you were straight and that you went to leather bars because you were not yet married and so you couldn't have sex with women?

AHMAD: Yes. I mean, I started going to leather bars by chance—right? And I found this wonderful place where I could have sex and stay anonymous. It was a revelation.

ME: But somewhere along the line you started to think that you were not straight, that you were bisexual.

AHMAD: Ya. I just assumed I was straight. I wasn't allowed to do much or see much growing up, so sex was a mystery. But I think about the leather bars a lot when I'm not going there. I think about having sex with men, even when my sex life is good with Layla. I know I'm bisexual.

ME: So growing up you weren't exposed to sexuality, or sex was secret . . .

AHMAD: Not talked about, not discussed. Not seen. Kids at school joked about stuff—but they didn't know any more than I did. And occasionally there would be a scandal, you know, in the papers, or people would gossip about people being in love and defying their families. Those stories never ended well.

ME: So, nothing about good sex, but it was joked about or you heard cautionary tales.

AHMAD: Lots of cautionary tales, little detail.

ME: That must have been hard.

AHMAD: No, not really. It was normal. And it seemed very doable—wait until marriage. I liked most parts of my life. I wish I hadn't been raised in what felt like a war zone, but I liked school, I liked prayer, I liked fasting, and feasting, I liked the order of things. Looking back, I really liked being around boys my age. I liked their bodies. I liked playing sports with them. I was turned on, but I didn't let myself know it.

ME: So your time in Palestine was both good and not good, and sexual and not sexual.

AHMAD: Good to be in a place where I felt like I belonged. Not good to be so confined and sometimes scared. And yes, good to be around good-looking boys, and maybe good that nothing ever came of it.

ME: What sexual outlets did you have? (*Ahmad shakes his head.*) What about masturbation?

AHMAD: Fast and furious. (*laughs*)

ME: What did you think about—what fantasies did you have?

AHMAD: I didn't think. If I would have thought, I probably would have thought I don't want my grandmother to find out, and since I didn't, don't, want to have my grandmother anywhere near my sexuality, I just did it quickly.

ME: Not much privacy.

AHMAD: No.

ME: So, what prompted you to masturbate when you did?

AHMAD: Oh, the crucial question. A cute boy? A cute girl?

ME: Or something else . . .

AHMAD: Well, there were no cute girls in my orbit. So yes, usually it was a boy that I thought about. But I also think I just needed a release, you know?

ME: So now, today, what do you think about when you masturbate?

AHMAD: I stand corrected. This is the crucial question. I think about guys.

ME: What do you make of that?

AHMAD: I enjoy sex with Layla. I do. But it is the sex I am supposed to have. Sex with men is supposed to be off-limits, so it's the sex I fantasize about.

ME: Isn't sex with other women off-limits too?

AHMAD: (*starting to get testy*) I only have Layla to think about because she is the only woman I've had sex with. I think about my experiences with men, my real-life experiences with men, when I masturbate.

ME: (*kindly*) Ahmad, I'm not questioning your sexuality. I'm trying to understand it. I keep hearing the same story from you—I like sex with men because . . . because it is the only option, because it is forbidden, because you have more memories. But really, don't you have sex with men and don't you think about sex with men because you find men sexually attractive and appealing?

AHMAD: Yes, yes, yes. I like sex with men. (*long pause*) I like sex with men more than I like sex with Layla. I don't want that to be true.

ME: Is it true?

AHMAD: Yes.

Ahmad did not like to think about sex. He did not question his sexual orientation; he did not let himself know he was attracted to boys, he did not fantasize during sex, and he did not want to consider that his attraction to men was stronger than his attraction to Layla. But I wanted Ahmad to think about his sexuality.

The culturally sensitive framework outlined by Hall and Graham (2020) entails exploring patients' sexuality within a cultural framework. This means understanding that culture partially determines the sexual experiences to which we have access, and that cultural messages also shape what we think and feel about those experiences. Ahmad may have innately had a stronger sexual attraction to men than he did to women. Bisexuality need not be a 50/50 proposition (Manley et al., 2015). But it is also possible that Ahmad's bisexuality was shaped by the fact of his uneven sexual history. Ahmad was able to have a lot of sex with men prior to his marriage, allowing him to explore and enjoy sex in that context. He felt free, anonymous, and without responsibility. His attraction to women had to be curtailed, and he was allowed to have sex with only one woman, his wife, who herself had no prior sexual experience.

So the "truth" that frightened Ahmad—which is that he is more attracted to men than to his wife—can be seen in a different light when viewed in cultural context. Ahmad's pleasurable sexual experiences with men far exceeded his opportunities to enjoy and even to fantasize about women. Furthermore, sex with his wife was his responsibility as her husband, and there were times when he just did not want to be responsible for one more thing. With this culturally informed hypothesis, I could continue to encourage Ahmad to think about and explore his sexuality.

ME: Ahmad, tell me what happens in the leather bars you go to.

AHMAD: (*obviously uncomfortable*) It's kind of hard to explain.

ME: No need to explain. Just describe what happens there. It's quite compelling to you, so it would help me to understand what happens there.

AHMAD: Uh, okay, well you know what a leather bar is, right?

ME: Ahmad, assume I know nothing about leather bars, which will be close to true.

The culturally sensitive framework encourages the therapist to become educated by the patient about their culture and sexuality, especially those aspects of their culture and sexuality of which the therapist is ignorant. I truly knew very little about the leather scene Ahmad was referencing. According to Ahmad, the leather bars or clubs he went to had several rooms or areas where scenes were performed. People could come and go as they chose, and may or may not participate in a certain scene. He often participated by being tied or otherwise constrained. He liked to be hit, spanked, and bitten, but he did not like sputum or urine or feces. He enjoyed oral sex (both giving and receiving), and he is a bottom—that is, he enjoyed receptive anal sex. He always practiced safe sex (required condoms in his scenes).

ME: You're very specific about what you like or want and what you don't.

AHMAD: It's all negotiated up front; as a lawyer, I like that. (*laughing*)

ME: So, what's it like for you when you're tied up—or down, as the case may be?

AHMAD: What's it like?

ME: Yes, what are you feeling—emotionally, physically . . . even spiritually, if that's relevant?

AHMAD: Emotionally? Not much. Happy maybe. Physically? Amazing.

ME: Amazing . . .

AHMAD: I don't know what's going to happen, but I trust absolutely that whatever happens, it will be for my pleasure. There's this exquisite balance of pain and pleasure and anticipation and satisfaction that makes me feel truly alive. And to know that others are watching—they're watching me—they're enjoying my pleasure and my pain and me. There is nothing better.

The culture of the leather scene that Ahmad rather poetically described also helps us understand his sexuality. We hear that at the leather bar, he "trusts," he feels "truly alive," he enjoys the fact that others are "enjoying his pleasure," and he feels there is "balance." I am not questioning his choices; questioning his preferences comes very close to pathologizing them. Listening and reflecting back, hallmarks of therapy, allowed Ahmad to explore his own sexuality more honestly. He came to appreciate the erotic appeal of trust, balance, and play in the sexual experience of feeling truly alive. He understood even more clearly why he was drawn to the leather bar. Ahmad talked about playing and feeling alive, in contrast to his adolescence, which had no play and a lot of fear of war and death. He talked about not having to be the responsible person in his sexual scenes, of the erotic appeal of trusting his pleasure to someone else. He talked about his admiration for the freedom he assumed the other men felt in walking clad in tight leather. He talked about how pain heightened his pleasure. Making assumptions about Ahmad's sexuality that are not reflected in his narrative (e.g., he likes the flogging because he is punishing himself) would be a distortion. The purpose of listening and reflecting is to encourage Ahmad to explore.

ME: So, we've talked about the complexity that your bisexuality adds to your life, but it sounds to me that sex with men is also kinky.

AHMAD: What do you mean?

ME: Pleasure, pain, bondage, that's what I mean by kink—what did you hear?

AHMAD: No, no, sorry. It's just that I know this must seem weird to you, and abnormal.

ME: (*gently*) Look, Ahmad. This is what I heard. I heard that you really enjoy the sex you have at the leather bar. I heard that you and everyone else involved consents, and that you practice safe sex, and that you really, really enjoy the sex you have there. You're here because you can't reconcile your sexual interests; you can't see how you can enjoy your bisexuality, and I'm wondering if you are also motivated to enjoy your interest in what I have called *kink*.

Ahmad was understandably sensitive to being judged for having sexual preferences that were not mainstream. As I described earlier in the chapter, individuals who enjoy power-based sexual practices such as BDSM, kink, and fetish often find that their sexual preferences are interpreted as signs of underlying psychopathology. This may explain why he did not explicitly identify his interests as kink. But as with his bisexuality, we can ask Ahmad about his sexual preferences without questioning or pathologizing them. Given that Ahmad hoped to be able to be happily monogamous, it was necessary to understand his sexual desires in order to see if he could reconcile his somewhat competing and conflicting sexual interests.

The culturally sensitive therapy model suggests that the process of acculturation can be applied to the process of psychotherapy. Acculturation occurs, to a greater or lesser extent, when two cultures meet, resulting in a blend or balance of elements from each. In this case, I offered Ahmad the opportunity to envision a merging of his two sexual worlds.

ME: Ahmad, have you ever asked Layla to tie you up, or to spank, pinch, or slap you during sex?

AHMAD: No. That's not an option.

ME: Why?

AHMAD: Trust me on this; it is not an option. Layla is a good woman. She's never had sex with anyone other than me, and she is always trying to do what is right.

ME: Giving you pleasure wouldn't be right?

AHMAD: Well, it would not be right to ask this of Layla, and if I did, she would also be more suspicious of me. I don't know, I don't know. Maybe that's what I need. A suspicious wife. Or a parole officer.

ME: (*laughing a little*) Sounds kinky.

AHMAD: (*laughing*) Thanks for that.

Actually, Ahmad is likely correct. It would not be right for him to ask things of Layla that she might not believe she has a right to refuse. Remember the message from Chapter 5 on desire: If you cannot say no, then yes has no meaning. Ahmad was in a conundrum. In a traditional marriage such as his, the husband is responsible and in charge. He could not know if Layla was acquiescing to his kink preferences because she is a good wife or if she was saying yes because she truly wanted to. The reverse may also be true. Layla might refuse, despite her interest in kink, because a good wife helps her husband maintain culturally correct sexual values. So, Ahmad could not be certain of her freedom to choose. In our therapeutic exploration, I wanted to reflect reality and imagine possibility; I wanted my work with Ahmad to lead to insights into how to bridge the cultural divide. Could heterosexual married sex also be kinky? Would that help Ahmad in his struggle to reconcile his competing sexual urges? Instead of possibilities, I was confronted with many of the obstacles that Ahmad experienced. And I could see and appreciate the difficulties he was encountering.

Ahmad's distress was palpable: "Help me. Help me stop going to leather bars. Please. This could ruin me." Our patients' distress always moves us. But often their distress is about something that cannot be quickly resolved. Ahmad initially hoped that therapy could help him eliminate or reduce his desire to go to leather bars. If this man—who survived being an American boy in Palestine and a Palestinian in America and who started his own law practice because he saw no future for himself at a big law firm—could not stop going to leather bars, then willpower was not the problem. I wanted to help Ahmad, and I wanted to help him quickly. I shared Ahmad's concern that he was on a collision course. But there are no sex therapy interventions or techniques that could do what Ahmad had originally hoped—to quickly reduce or eliminate his desire to go to leather bars. Therapy was helpful to Ahmad because he felt less isolated. He felt understood: We were in this together.

A Not-So-Happy Ending

Time and luck did run out for Ahmad. Layla found pictures Ahmad had taken of himself in his leather gear. She left him. She took their children. A family court judge granted Ahmad only supervised visits with his children after his wife used the pictures as evidence against his parental fitness. Unfortunately, Ahmad's experience is not unique; people's sexual preferences and behaviors are often used against them in child custody cases.

Ahmad became very depressed. Therapy was a safe place to crash and pick up the pieces. His mother and brothers stood by him and said that if he was gay, they were okay with that. He was too shattered to tell them that he was not gay. That would wait for later. Meanwhile, he found himself ostracized by many in his community, only to be befriended by others who felt that Ahmad's wife was duty bound to return home and who therefore wanted to help Ahmad forcefully bring his wife and children back. Luckily, Ahmad resisted those overtures.

After his separation, Ahmad went on a bit of a sex bender, to borrow from the addiction lexicon. He had a lot of sex with a lot of men and briefly dated a man. But he found himself longing for a monogamous marriage with a wife, a family, and Muslim traditions and values. He dated a few American women who were open to raising their children as Muslim, but Ahmad really wanted a Muslim wife. Being divorced and the focus of gossip, he was not the prize husband he once was. Paradoxically, this freed Ahmad from matchmakers and allowed him to choose a wife for himself. Ultimately, Ahmad did remarry. He married a Muslim American woman who was divorced. She knew about his bisexuality and his interest in kink because he told her upfront. He did not want to hide himself in this marriage. She was open to exploring kink but struggled with Ahmad's bisexuality, worried that he would inevitably cheat on her with a man.

Therapy helped Ahmad balance and integrate his two sexual worlds (a conscious process of acculturation), rather than keeping them separate. Presently, he masturbates to gay fantasies and porn. His sex life with Gigi (his wife) sometimes includes light restraints, sex toys, and mild impact play (slapping, biting, and pinching). It is fun and playful, and Gigi brought her own sexual experiences to enhance their sexual repertoire.

Is this a happy ending? Maybe. It is a compromise. It is a resolution that brought relief to Ahmad's mother and brothers. In many ways, it brought relief to Ahmad. He was able to obtain joint custody of his children, and he regained the respect of his religious community. But this outcome came at a cost that Ahmad bore in private. He is still not reconciled to never having sex with another man and never again going to a leather bar. He holds out some hope that he may renegotiate the boundaries of his relationship with Gigi so that he may, under certain circumstances, again enjoy his kink preferences with a man. Ahmad has continued in therapy. He finds it helpful to navigate through his life with therapy, which is the one place where he can be fully himself and talk openly about his bisexuality and his kink.

SUMMARY

A lot has changed over the years in how we view paraphilias or kink. We now understand that sexual minority patients are not much different from other patients who consult with us regarding their fears and thwarted desires. The lack of evidence linking an interest in kink to underlying psychopathology has led the *DSM* to eliminate the diagnosis of paraphilia and instead only diagnose paraphilic disorder in those instances where there is coercion or lack of consent, or if the patient experiences distress or impairment in their life. Therapists know how to treat people who are distressed because they do not live up to familial or sociocultural standards, so therapists have the skills to help kinky people who experience distress and impairment. The clinical focus needs to be on the distress and impairment, not on the sex.

A culturally sensitive approach to sex therapy is a helpful model for working with sexual minority patients in that it helps shift the focus from individual pathology to an exploration of the cultural influences that have shaped sexual interests and contributed to sexual distress. The culturally sensitive sex therapy approach emphasizes the need for listening with exquisite sensitivity and without judgment to the patient's experience and provides a path for the integration of sexual desires rather than focusing on the futile endeavor of ridding the patient of them.

8 SEXUAL ISSUES IN COUPLES THERAPY

As a young child, I used to angle the two mirrors hanging in our bathroom to simultaneously see multiple images of myself. The number of images formed when two mirrors are inclined toward each other depends on the angle between them. Infinite reflections are possible (Vedantu, 2024). When colored pieces of glass or other opaque material are enclosed in a tube containing angled mirrors, a kaleidoscope is formed. Consider this an analogy for the chaotic, colorful process that is couples therapy.

In individual therapy, there is one person who commands the therapist's attention. In couples therapy, it is not so straightforward. In couples therapy, therapists have to simultaneously attend to the couple in front of them and each of the two individuals making up that couple while also focusing on the relationship those two individuals have with each other. A couples therapist, like an individual therapist, still has to pay attention to the therapeutic relationship; however, in the case of couples therapy, this means having an awareness of the dynamic between the therapist and each member of the couple, as well as the dynamic between the couple (as a unit) and the therapist. It is no wonder then that couples therapy is both exhausting and exhilarating. This chapter explores how to talk about sex in the chaotic, colorful process of couples therapy.

https://doi.org/10.1037/0000483-009
Talking About Sex in Psychotherapy: A Guide for Every Therapist, by K. S. K. Hall

WHO IS RIGHT? WHICH STORY IS MORE REAL?

In childhood, when I was confronted with multiple reflections in the mirror, I wondered which image was the closest approximation to how I truly looked. Which one was me? In other words, I wanted to know which of the many reflections was the most real. In couples therapy, we are not engaged with this question of "most real." Many, if not all, of the viewpoints are valid. The process of couples therapy requires working with multiple perspectives, which can be helpfully incorporated into a new view of the relationship.

Couple constellations differ. Made up of two people, couples may be of the same or different genders, ages, ethnicities, and religions. Some couplings involve a merging or submerging of individual identities, whereas others place a greater emphasis on the maintenance of individuality. Some therapists have noted the inverse relationship between lust and enmeshed domesticity (Morin, 1995; Perel, 2006), observing that obstacles and distance increase desire. Arranged marriages are built on the understanding that a sexual union develops from shared values and purpose within the marriage, whereas love marriages rely on preexisting sexual attractions upon which to base their sexual relationship.

While we are looking at the kaleidoscope of images presented to us by the couple in therapy, they of course are looking at us: How are we reacting and responding to them and to their partner? For example, one patient, Tim, challenged me early on in therapy by asking me why I more often looked toward his wife, Nancy, when I was talking. What I learned from his question was that (a) he was keeping track; (b) he was in competition with his wife for my attention; (c) he felt left out, disregarded, and dismissed; and (d) he was unaware of the signals he was putting out that were putting me off (and likely others too). I told Tim that I had not been aware I was favoring his wife in general but would pay more attention to that in the future. I also told him that I did know, in this moment, that I was directing my attention to Nancy. I told him that his wife was smiling and nodding, thereby letting me know that she wanted to hear what I was saying, whereas he was scowling at me. Tim was satisfied with the answer. It was honest, and it gave us something we could work on. It made Tim aware of a behavior that likely turned many people away from him.

My interaction with Tim also had an impact on Nancy, as it inevitably would (after all, she was there with us). I wondered aloud about her reaction. She responded that she was all too familiar with Tim's negativity—toward herself and toward others. I asked her whether she felt that she needed to be more engaging and supportive than she sometimes felt to balance out her husband's negativity. When Nancy said she thought that was true, Tim turned to her and said, "I really hate it when you do that." She paused, held back the defensive retort that usually came when she felt criticized, and instead said, "Me too." Perhaps Nancy was able to answer Tim as she did because she witnessed my nondefensive response to her husband's criticism (and his acceptance of it) and therefore saw a new possibility. Or perhaps, being in therapy, she was just ready to make some changes.

The individuals who make up the couple in the therapy room will often want the therapist to determine who is right or wrong, whose feelings are justified or not; in other words, they are asking the question I asked of the mirrors—which reflection is real? When the topic is sex, the questions often turn to "Is this okay? Normal? Weird? Are my responses acceptable? Understandable?" These questions take on added depth because it is not often, if ever, that couples reveal their sexual relationship fully to another person. The opportunity to explore their sexual relationship with a caring and compassionate therapist is a rare gift of therapy.

It is my contention that a couple's sex life, even if it is nonexistent, is possibly the best window into the intimate workings of their relationship. To explore this idea in more depth and also to see the impact of multiple mirrors on the process of therapy, I offer the case of Jan and Zofia, a couple married for 26 years, who immigrated to the United States from their native Poland about 7 years prior to my first meeting them.

JAN AND ZOFIA

At the time that Jan (pronounced "Yaan") and Zofia came to therapy, they had not had sex in either 2 years or 6 months, depending on whom you were talking to. According to Zofia, the lack of sex for the last 6 months related to her anger over Jan's infidelity. According to Jan, there was no sex prior to his seeking sex elsewhere, and the lack of sex in his marriage over the last 2 years more than justified his having sex outside his marriage. Furthermore, as he patiently explained to me, what he did not count as infidelity, given that he only had sex with sex workers and he only did it when he was on business back in their native Poland.

Both Jan and Zofia wanted to preserve the marriage, citing the importance of their family, their finances, and their place within the Polish expat community. This was about all they agreed upon. Jan was adamant that he did nothing wrong, and he thought that the problem was that Zofia was becoming too American, being frequently argumentative and withholding sex, which she had never done prior to emigrating. Jan often interrupted therapy to explain to me the cultural importance of his viewpoint—"In Poland . . ."; "According to our traditions . . ."; and "What you don't understand is . . ."—leading up to his inevitable conclusion that Polish wives do not withhold sex. To do so is a violation of trust, a betrayal of marital vows and traditions, and an affront to his masculinity and his role in the family—and it more than justifies extramarital sex. Zofia disagreed. Infidelity, according to her, was and is wrong in whatever country or context it occurs. Furthermore, she did not refuse to have sex with Jan; she refused to have sex with Jan when she did not feel like it, when she was tired or unwell.

I reflected back to the couple their differing views on their marriage: "So, you have not had sex in a while; it has been somewhere between 6 months and 2 years, and since that time your relationship has changed. This change, this decrease or absence of sex, has been primarily directed by Zofia." Thus, Jan and Zofia each felt heard, and each felt that I was not taking sides. The fact that the therapist can hold multiple perspectives without judgment on contentious subjects such as sex is both vital to the process of therapy and reassuring to the couple.

Jan has also added a cultural perspective to the therapy process through his frequent references to their Polish background. The culturally sensitive lens (Hall & Graham, 2014, 2020) discussed in Chapter 7 entails listening closely to sexual stories without preconceived judgments. It is essentially good clinical practice when working with all patients, regardless of the extent to which they appear more or less similar to our own cultural backgrounds. Jan presented ideas about sex and marriage that are likely to be disagreeable to the majority of Western-trained therapists. He could easily be viewed as entitled, misogynistic, and narcissistic. And he may be all these things, hiding behind a culturally inspired rationalization, but I at least needed to try to see his marriage from his vantage point before I could work with him.

Jan and Zofia had immigrated for financial reasons, hoping to earn enough money to live well and send money back to Poland to care for their aging parents. They also wanted their three children to attend university in the United States. Jan had been the main wage earner in Poland, but in the United States, it was Zofia who landed the better-paying, high-level job in a reputable investment firm. Two years previously, Zofia was promoted to a challenging new position, managing a team and having responsibility for a large financial portfolio. She was often tired by the end of the week. Jan wanted to have sex on Friday evening, as was their custom—to have sex on Friday evening,

Saturday, and Sunday, with no sex during the work week, as Jan often commuted long distances for various consulting jobs. Zofia began to refuse sex on Friday, claiming fatigue. Soon they were having sex on Saturday and often (but not always) on Sunday. To Jan, this decrease in frequency counted as no sex. Jan took frequent trips back to Poland to visit his aging parents and to take care of their financial interests. During these trips, he hired sex workers. Because they were sex workers and because it was far from the marital home in the United States, this could not be construed as wrong according to Jan; it could and should be seen as a husband trying his best to stay faithful to a wife who was neglecting her marriage. Zofia discovered Jan's activities when she was notified by their credit card company of potentially fraudulent charges.

If I had seen Jan and Zofia prior to the infidelity, they would have been a couple who presented with a desire discrepancy. Jan wanted sex three times a week, whereas Zofia would have been happy with once, maybe twice a week. Desire discrepancies are frequent complaints that couples have about sex—how often is enough? Do you need a "good" reason not to have sex? Do you need a good reason to have sex? Jan thought that Zofia's tiredness was not a good reason to refuse sex. He was upset that she was not interested in being with him sexually after a hectic work week. Zofia interpreted Jan's interest in sex as selfish because it disregarded her fatigue after a hectic work week. Jan's desire for sex was not a good enough reason for having sex with him, according to the more American version of Zofia.

Couples often argue about frequency because it is an objective measure of something more intangible: "I don't feel desirable. I don't believe that you desire me." It is my clinical experience, shared by many of my colleagues, that couples who present to therapy with desire discrepancy related to how often they were or were not having sex sometimes leave therapy very happy with their sex life, despite an unchanged frequency, or even a lower frequency, of sex. It is the quality of sex and the mutual feeling of being desired that is the happy outcome they had not been able to articulate prior to therapy. (Of course, greater satisfaction can and often does lead to having more frequent sex, so some couples do leave therapy having sex more often than they once did.)

The difference between three times a week and twice may not feel like a significant differential to us, but it felt very significant for Jan. Other desire-discrepant couples present with more obvious margins between what they each want regarding sexual frequency. The most difficult cases of discrepancy are those in which one partner does not want to have sex at all and the other does. To digress from Jan and Zofia for a moment, we can consider another couple struggling with desire discrepancy.

GAIL AND FRANK

Gail, a 60-year-old woman, asked, "Don't couples live happily together with no sex?" "Yes," I replied, "but they only live happily if both partners agree." In Gail's case, her husband, Frank, was deeply troubled by Gail's lack of interest in sex. They used to have an active sex life, but the frequency of sex had dwindled over the years from twice a week to about once a month. Neither was happy with this. For Frank, it was not often enough, while Gail did not want any sex at all.

Gail and Frank had fallen into a trap that many couples find themselves in: Gail avoided any physical or intimate contact with Frank for fear it would lead to sex. Frank thought that on those rare occasions when there was some affectionate contact, he should see if Gail might be open to having sex. When sex did not happen, Frank would feel hurt and rejected, and he would withdraw physically and emotionally from Gail. "He only ever touches me when he wants sex. He's never affectionate. He only wants sex," is how Gail thought about these interactions, so she renewed her efforts to avoid intimate and physical contact. Their marriage was becoming devoid of affection and intimacy, making sex an ever more remote possibility.

In these two mirrors, one reflected an aging man whose sexuality was vitally important to him as he wanted to fully embrace life and his connection to Gail before it was too late. The second mirror reflected a woman tired of taking care of others, who wanted to use her time and energy, now freed from taking care of children, for herself. These mirrors were not inclined toward each other, so infinite possibilities were not reflected back. It was my job as their therapist to position these mirrors so that Frank and Gail could see each other and understand each other's perspective.

Many therapists would want to explore the reasons behind Gail's disinterest—lack of love or buried resentments, perhaps? It is rare for the motivations of the higher-desiring partner to be questioned, reflecting the bias that desire is normal and lack of desire is not. But Frank's reasons for desire were as important as Gail's feelings. So, I asked Frank what kept his interest in having sex with Gail alive? With encouragement, Frank talked about his loneliness and his sadness about aging and losing what passion time still allowed him; he talked about wanting intimate contact with Gail, cuddling, hugging, and kissing, not just sex (but yes, also sex).

Frank heard Gail speak about the stress she felt when she knew he wanted sex, how hard it was to know she was letting him down, and how she would resolve each day that she would have sex with him, but the resolve for the day would turn into a promise for tomorrow and would never happen. Gail knew that their lives were stalled as the unresolved question of sex hung between them.

"When did you first notice a change in your sex life? When do you think your desires started to diverge?" I asked. Both agreed that in retrospect, there were problems dating back 10 years, which Gail identified as the time she was going through menopause. "What was it about menopause that interfered with sex?" I asked. Some women attribute changes to hormones, others to a change in their physical appearance, while some talk about other co-occurring life events, such as the empty nest or retirement from work. Many women, Gail included, noted that intercourse became painful. According to the North American Menopause Society (n.d.a), reduced levels of estrogen cause the tissues of the vulva and the lining of the vagina to become thinner, drier, and less elastic or flexible (collectively referred to as vulvovaginal atrophy). Vaginal secretions during sexual stimulation are also reduced. These now drier and more fragile vulvovaginal tissues are susceptible to injury (tearing, bleeding). The vagina may also become shorter and narrower if penetrative sex does not occur on a regular basis, and then intercourse is likely to be painful, even when a lubricant is used.

Intercourse was painful for Gail postmenopause, which Frank knew, and that was why he was not asking for penetrative sex. But instead of Gail being relieved, she felt burdened; with little or no sexual desire, engaging in sex without the option of intercourse required a lot more effort on her part. This is something Gail would never have said to Frank without the nonjudgmental questioning and affirmation she got from therapy. "It is a lot more effort," I responded. Frank sat glumly by, watching two women commiserate on how much work it was to have sex (and one of them was talking about how much work it was to have sex with him). I said to Frank, "What's it like to hear that?" He shrugged.

ME: Gail, what was it like to say that aloud?

GAIL: It was hard. I don't want to hurt his feelings, and I don't want to sound selfish, but I just can't go on pretending.

FRANK: I don't want you to pretend.

ME: So if perhaps sex was a little less effortful on your part, Gail, and somehow more enjoyable, it would be better for both of you.

In a subsequent session, Gail happily reported that Frank had given her a long backrub and that she reciprocated by caressing his chest and legs while Frank masturbated to orgasm. Over the next few months, they explored other ways to make sex more enjoyable for both of them, understanding that since Frank wanted to have sex more than Gail did, he would need to put in a bit more effort to make sex happen, and they would both also need to become more comfortable enjoying nonsexual affectionate intimacy (despite the unspoken question of whether this would turn into sex). Previously, Frank had told Gail that he would wait for her to initiate sex because he was tired of being rejected. But this was another losing strategy. It created tension, with Gail resenting that she had to be responsible for sex that she did not even want. It also led to Frank impatiently waiting for Gail to initiate, building his frustration, resentment, and hurt.

During the course of therapy, Gail and Frank scheduled time to be together. They did not schedule time for sex (that would be obligation). But they needed to set aside time to be together, a time when sex might be possible if they felt so inclined. Many couples think that sex should be spontaneous, but with busy lives, there might not be many opportunities. Often, having sex at the end of the day, when all other pleasures and chores are done, does not leave much energy for it. Recent research confirms my clinical experience that planned sex is just as pleasurable as spontaneous sex (Kovacevic et al., 2024). I often use the analogy of going to a restaurant. You make reservations in advance. Once there, you look at the menu and choose the food you feel like eating in the moment. A time when sex is possible can be planned. What you do in the moment will be driven by what you desire in the moment. We can think back to Basson's (2001) circular model of sexual response outlined in Chapter 1. Sex can be driven by the desire for closeness or the anticipation of pleasure, or as happened during the backrubs, desire can follow arousal rather than having to precede it.

The backrubs were sometimes enjoyed on their own, and sometimes they led to sex. When Frank wanted sex, the backrubs were a lot more sensual, and when Gail was open to sex, she encouraged the sensual touch with body language and soft moans of pleasure. The sex that followed the backrubs varied. Sometimes Gail stimulated Frank with her hand or performed fellatio; sometimes she would masturbate, or Frank would stimulate her to orgasm with his hand (she did not want oral sex). But the pressure to have sex as they had in the past was gone, and Frank and Gail found a way to be sexual that worked for them both. The frequency of sex was about once a month, a frequency they had both initially rejected but now enjoyed.

I did suggest to Gail that if she was interested in resuming intercourse, she could consult with her gynecologist about hormone therapy and also use vaginal dilators to help restore vaginal elasticity. But Gail talked it over with Frank, and they decided that they were happy with the frequency and quality of the sex they were now enjoying.

RETURNING TO JAN AND ZOFIA

I met Jan and Zofia, not when they were struggling with how often to have sex, but only after Zofia's discovery of Jan's extramarital sexual activity. Much to Jan's chagrin, his infidelity was the initial focus of therapy rather than the lower frequency of sex, which he felt was the real problem. This is often, if not always, the case when infidelity occurs in an agreed-upon monogamous relationship. Infidelity and its fallout become the primary focus of treatment. How this is accomplished differs according to how infidelity is conceptualized. When infidelity is viewed as a betrayal or an attachment injury, as it frequently is, treatment strategies emphasize the need to heal the injury first (Fife et al., 2023; Warach & Josephs, 2021). The dark triad of personality traits (narcissism, Machiavellianism, psychopathy) frequently associated with unfaithful partners directs the therapist's attention to those characterological problems (Josephs, 2018, Chapter 4; see also Josephs, 2020).

Jan's frequent references to his Polish roots served as a reminder of the relevance of culture. Most of the research on infidelity comes from white, heterosexual, cisgender North American samples (Weiser et al., 2023). A wider cultural lens is needed to truly understand many of the nuances of infidelity and the context in which it occurs. Esther Perel, a Belgian-born psychotherapist, interviewed hundreds of people who had experienced infidelity (including the transgressor, the transgressed, and the other), and she consulted with therapists, philosophers, and sex researchers. In her resulting book, *The State of Affairs* (Perel, 2017), Perel presents the intriguing hypothesis that some people cheat to reclaim a past and forgotten part of themselves. Perel encourages the reader to look beyond the apparently selfish motivation of the person having an affair to see instead a person who has longing and desire. And that desire may not be for another person but for the self they once were. In light of Perel's hypothesis, the fact that Jan hired sex workers only when he returned to Poland, the country where he had once felt like an important person, is likely very relevant for understanding his motivation.

Focusing on Sex

Notwithstanding the hurt often caused by emotional affairs, what we typically think about when infidelity is mentioned is sex. For Jan and Zofia, it was all about the sex. Jan hired sex workers with whom he did not form any romantic or intimate connection. In fact, he never (knowingly) hired the same sex worker twice. The transgression was sexual. Zofia expressed her anger and hurt by withholding sex from her husband. (She continued to cook for him, eat meals together, socialize with their friends, and participate in family activities.) The battleground was sex. After 6 months of trying to work things out on their own, and then almost 2 months in therapy, they were at a stalemate characterized, on the one hand, by Jan's insistence that sex should resume since he had done nothing wrong and, on the other hand, by Zofia's insistence on an apology, an explanation, and a commitment to monogamy before there would be any sex.

I would argue that if sex is the battleground, then therapy needs to start there. The three mirrors that are relevant are Jan and Zofia's separate perspectives on their sexual relationship and Jan's perspective on the sex he had with sex workers. Talking about sex with individuals is one thing; talking about it with couples is another. In most if not all cases, I ask couples about their mutual sex life when they are together, but then I also schedule individual sessions to explore more deeply. This allows each person to amend their observations once they do not need to worry about their partner's feelings and reactions, and also once they have hopefully built some trust in me (that I am not judgmental and that I will listen).

Harkening all the way back to Chapter 4, on shame and secrets, it is important to give people the opportunity to reveal themselves more honestly as therapy progresses. Shame abounds around sex, and it thrives in cases of infidelity. Often, but not always, the person who had the extramarital sex feels shame (I am a cheater. How could I have hurt the person I love? How could I give up my affair partner when I care so deeply for them?), and the person who was cheated on feels shame (How could I not have known? Why don't I have the self-esteem to leave? Why was this done to me? What is wrong with me?). Zofia and Jan, however, were so angry with each other that they could not initially share any sense of shame with each other, making the task of reconciliation more difficult. Zofia's shame was deeper than the infidelity; she wondered why she had married Jan in the first place, and she desperately needed his shame to reassure her that staying with him was not weakness on her part. Jan's shame was also about more than the infidelity. He had few emotional resources to cope with the displacement he felt upon immigrating to the United States. He felt shame about his lack of success, especially compared to Zofia's career trajectory. He could not admit that he was wrong to have had extramarital sex.

Secrets and Lies in Couples Therapy

When Zofia had her individual session with me, I told her quite directly the same thing I had told Jan:

> This session is about you, your perspectives on your marriage, on your sexual relationship with Jan, and on the infidelity. It is likely that some of your answers will differ from the ones we talked about when Jan was present. In this session, your perspective is the only one I am interested in. What you say in the session with me today is between the two of us. If it is something that would be important to talk about with Jan, we can discuss whether and when and how to do that. That would be a decision you would make with my help. What you say to me will be confidential. I won't discuss with Jan what you have told me here today. And I have told the same thing to Jan.

This is essentially a reiteration of what Jan and Zofia already knew about how I worked, but it never hurts to repeat information about boundaries. I promised each of them that what they told me in their individual sessions would have the same degree of confidentiality that they could be assured of in individual therapy.

Couples therapists have a conflicted relationship with secrets. We want our patients to tell us everything. We count on them to tell us the truth, as therapy is predicated upon truth. In return for truth, we promise strict confidentiality, a safe place for secrets to be held and processed. This is our agreement with patients in individual therapy. But when it comes to couples therapy, we are reluctant to offer the same confidentiality to the individuals who make up the couple. Watter (2022) outlined three models for couples sex therapy:

1. There is no allowance for individual communications from either partner; everything that is known to the therapist is known to both members of the couple.

2. Individual sessions may occur with the stipulation that whatever is shared in those sessions will be shared in the couple's sessions. Thus, there is no confidentiality promised to the individual.

3. Individual sessions may occur with a guarantee of confidentiality. Thus, there is the potential for the therapist to hold a secret with one (or both) member(s) of the couple.

The discomfort that many therapists have with this third model is that it raises the possibility of collusion and harm for at least one person in the couple relationship. It is also a very tricky balance for a therapist to maintain. Watter (2022) clarifies his preference for this third model because he believes it is best to know all the issues at play when working with a couple. Watter tells couples who are uncomfortable with these boundaries that they may choose a different therapist with a different approach—although in his 40-plus years of clinical practice, this has happened to him only once (Watter, personal communication, September 8, 2023). In this third approach, which allows for confidentiality, the therapist can still be balanced and unbiased, and can still maintain the goal of helping the couple, even if and when the therapist holds a secret. Ethical practice requires the couple's consent to whatever model is practiced.

Therapists worry most that if they promise confidentiality, an ongoing affair will be revealed in an individual session, which will put them in an awkward situation or render couples therapy moot. Infidelity is only one possible secret. Other sexual secrets may be attractions, interests, faked orgasms, masturbation habits, and fantasies. Other nonsexual secrets may include finances, friendships, and emotions. I would argue that the content of the secret may not be as important as the function of the secret.

Jan and Zofia did indeed have secrets from each other. Zofia told me in an individual session that she had long felt sexually unsatisfied by Jan. Getting a vibrator helped. But she had found it increasingly tedious to stimulate him to an erection, and she wondered whether he was having erection problems. It was not something she felt she could ask him. Another secret was that she had developed an emotional relationship with someone at work but had broken it off before she found out about Jan's infidelity, and she was now regretting that decision, as the person in question was now in a committed relationship with someone else. Zofia was keeping two secrets for slightly different reasons. The first secret, about her sexual unhappiness, was kept to maintain the relationship status quo (based on her understanding of two dynamics: that Jan had a fragile sense of self, which could not tolerate perceived criticism, and also that her needs were secondary to his).

The second secret, about the emotional relationship, was initially kept to preserve the marriage, but now it was kept for the additional purpose of maintaining a moral edge over Jan. She could say to herself, "I never cheated. I am not a selfish person. I gave up love for you, whereas you couldn't hold back on having meaningless sex for me. I am the good person. You are the bad person here." If Zofia had said this aloud, it is likely that the secret may have had a different resonance. Jan may have countered, "You also cheated in letting that relationship go so far; what you did is worse because you cared about someone else." Wanting to keep a moral high ground is not an unusual stance for someone who has historically had less power in a relationship. Secrets can be powerful, and holding them can confer power. Zofia wanted to preserve the moral high ground, but a moral high ground is not often a place of growth.

I wondered whether Jan had other affairs during his marriage to Zofia. If he had, he never revealed it to me in individual sessions or to Zofia. He had tried to keep his now-known interactions with sex workers a secret from Zofia for two reasons: (a) he wanted to remain married to Zofia; and (b) he wanted to regain a sense of his former self, the self-assured and successful Polish businessman, not the business consultant struggling with English and hustling for clients (note that the first explanation was his stated reason and the second was my clinical opinion). Individual sessions with Jan were spent discussing his interactions with sex workers, something that would have been hurtful for Zofia to participate in, and her participation would have interfered with Jan's ability to be honest. But the devil is sometimes in the details, and I wanted to know if my assumption about his desire to feel important was a helpful interpretation.

As he described the sex he had, it was nothing particularly kinky or different from the sex he had with Zofia. What he tended to like the most was specifying which woman he wanted, and he liked the expressions of interest and appreciation they voiced during his time with them. Jan said he knew that they were "likely not true" and "probably done to get me to cum quicker," but "it worked. It turned me on." He added, "But if they were trying to get me to be a repeat customer, that didn't work." So, overall, it did seem that Jan was playing out a power dynamic to feel superior in his sexual interactions with sex workers. At least it was a reasonable hypothesis, which later in therapy Jan himself identified.

Jan and Zofia essentially agreed on what their sex life together had been like. Not surprisingly, their descriptions depicted sexual interactions centered on Jan's needs. Essentially, sex happened on Jan's timetable (hence the weekend schedule), and the initiation of sex was something like Jan asking Zofia, "Are you ready to go to bed now?" They each undressed and got into bed. Foreplay consisted of Zofia fondling Jan's penis and performing fellatio until he had a firm erection. Jan would fondle Zofia's breasts and rub her genitals until she was lubricated (wet). Jan would then decide that it was time to have intercourse, which they did with Jan thrusting for several minutes until he ejaculated. Thus satisfied, Jan would roll over and sleep, or head to the bathroom to clean himself.

Things changed slightly when, several years ago, Zofia purchased a vibrator and used it to stimulate herself to orgasm once Jan ejaculated. Jan claimed to be happy that Zofia had found the vibrator helpful, but he noted that his other lovers prior to marriage had not needed such devices and had had orgasms during intercourse. He surmised, incorrectly, that there was something wrong with Zofia that she needed a vibrator. Zofia was pleased to be having orgasms during partnered sex, even if Jan was sometimes not even in the room. Jan was her first and only sex partner, and she believed him when he told her that she should be having orgasms when they had intercourse. Apart from the addition of the vibrator, their sex life had remained virtually unchanged during their 26 years together, and there was little to no variety in how they had sex from one time to the next.

Jan was wrong to think that Zofia should be having orgasms from intercourse alone. I needed to correct this misinformation as it was important. But I was mindful not to add to Jan's sense of shame. What I said was this:

> You know, the idea that women should have orgasms from intercourse was an idea that Freud really promoted. But until recently, no one knew much about the anatomy and physiology of the clitoris. So, it wasn't until the late 1990s that physicians discovered that the clitoris is not just that little button-like structure where the labia meet, but it actually has legs that extend down, sometimes as far as the vagina, and they extend around the vaginal opening. So, some women can have orgasms from the thrusting of intercourse alone. But actually, most women need that little button structure—otherwise known as the head of the clitoris—to be stimulated for an orgasm to occur (see Appendix A for a more detailed description of the clitoris and orgasm).

Zofia was really interested, and I directed them both to Laurie Mintz's (2017) book *Becoming Cliterate*, in which she discusses the pleasure gap (Herbenick et al., 2018). The gap refers to the fact that in heterosexual sexual interactions, men are more likely to experience pleasure and orgasm compared to their female partners. One reason for the orgasm gap is that the direct clitoral stimulation that results in orgasm when women masturbate is rarely replicated in partnered sex. Some men, like Jan, mistakenly assume that women should orgasm during intercourse as men do. And many women feel self-conscious that they are "taking too much time" to reach orgasm, so they do not ask for the stimulation they might need, or they fake an orgasm so that their partner will be simultaneously gratified and will stop trying (Herbenick et al., 2019).

Deconstructing Sex

We can learn a lot from taking a dispassionate view—in other words, taking a step back and looking at the sexual relationship that Jan and Zofia had forged over the years. One striking observation is how little desire there was. Sex was routinized to fit into Jan's work schedule. It was an obligation. The initiation of sex was devoid of expressions of actual interest: "Are you ready to go to bed now?" There was no flirting, no kissing, no fondling, and no kindling of desire or excitement. Zofia and Jan agreed that their sexual activities invariably happened in the same sequence and had for the past 26 years. When sex is so routinized, something other than lust is driving the decisions. No wonder neither Jan nor Zofia felt desired by the other—they had eliminated desire from sex.

Jan and Zofia agreed that sex changed when Zofia got a promotion at work and was too tired for the usual Friday night sex. But encouraged to think a little more about it, Zofia also said that she started to question what was happening sexually between them when she starting watching the television shows that her friends at work were talking about. Often the shows alluded to the sexual pleasure that the female characters were experiencing, and sometimes they openly discussed orgasms and vibrators, which prompted Zofia to buy a vibrator of her own. She masturbated for the first time at 47 years of age. And for the first time in her life, Zofia experienced orgasm. So, in addition to Zofia making more money and being more professionally successful, Jan sought sex outside the marriage when Zofia began to have orgasms with the vibrator (and not with Jan's participation). The introduction of the vibrator was a narcissistic injury to Jan, not a fun and helpful sex toy. He responded to Zofia's orgasms as he did to her career success: with jealousy and hurt. Zofia was not going to relinquish her career success, and I was hopeful that I could help this couple rebalance their sex life so that Zofia would not have to relinquish or relegate her pleasure to a secondary status.

Both Jan and Zofia were dissatisfied with their sex life. Jan's dissatisfaction led him to seek out sex workers, but the transactional nature of the sex he paid for was a continuation of his opting for obligation over desire. This older, educated couple seemed unable to navigate a mutually pleasurable sex life for themselves, despite 26 years together and traveling halfway across the world to make a new life.

Their inability to resolve their differences presaged a crisis in therapy. Several months into the therapy, Zofia was still refusing to have sex with Jan until he apologized and took responsibility for his infidelity, and Jan was still refusing to do so. One evening, Jan insisted on sex. Zofia still refused. This went on for several hours, with Jan insisting and Zofia refusing. She locked herself in the bedroom, and Jan broke down the door. Zofia, fearful, taunted Jan: "Go ahead and do it." As he touched her, Zofia stiffened and, luckily, Jan stopped. They called for an emergency session. They were now frightened enough to change.

SEXUAL VIOLENCE: CONTRAINDICATIONS TO COUPLES THERAPY

Not all difficulties, not all people, and not all relationships are suitable for psychotherapy. Some people struggle with honesty in couples therapy because they know there will be consequences (arguing, the silent treatment, or physical abuse) once they are outside the therapy office and back at home. Couples therapy cannot and should not occur when there is not a reasonable expectation of safety. Couples therapists often set boundaries regarding discussions outside of therapy to minimize the possibility of repercussions for honest participation in the therapy process. Sex therapists also set boundaries to help couples navigate problematic sex such that the risk of abuse and coercion is mitigated. In these cases, what is safe and permissible is negotiated and agreed to in therapy, with the therapist checking in during subsequent sessions to monitor compliance with boundaries. Either therapy is terminated, or the focus of therapy is changed to address safety concerns when patients do not or cannot adhere to reasonable limits.

In many cultures, women simply do not have the right to refuse sex with their husbands, and attempting to do so can result in sexual violence. It was not until 1993 that all 50 states across the United States abolished the marital exception to recognize marital rape as a crime (Brown et al., 2020). Still, the differences in marital and nonmarital rape statutes render marital rape much harder to prosecute, with some states still offering some form of marital immunity, and with legal consequences typically being much less severe in comparison to nonmarital rape. Rape, or aggravated sexual abuse (the correct legal terminology), is defined as using force or the threat of force to cause another person to engage in a sexual act. But the myths that abound regarding intimate partner or marital rape serve to trivialize the offense. These myths include the belief that being raped by an intimate partner is less traumatic than being raped by a stranger, that spouses or partners will leave if they have been raped, and that husbands are just asserting their right to sex and therefore their behavior cannot be construed as rape (Lilley et al., 2023).

Sexual violence also occurs in dating and other relationship constellations (Fernet et al., 2021; Jeffrey & Barata, 2021). Keilholtz and Spencer (2022) outlined factors to include in assessments (conducted with partners seen separately) as well as a list of helpful assessment instruments for use in situations of intimate partner violence.

When one partner uses violence to intimidate, control, or gain power over the other, couples therapy is generally contraindicated. This does not include therapeutic programs specifically targeting intimate partner violence (Keilholtz & Spencer, 2022). I have similarly argued that sex therapy is contraindicated in relationships where there is a significant power imbalance between partners such that one partner does not have the right to consent or to withhold consent for sexual activities (Hall, 2019). Psychotherapy for couples is predicated upon a reasonably equitable degree of safety and autonomy.

RETURNING TO JAN AND ZOFIA

Jan and Zofia were engaged in a struggle for power. They came to see me for an emergency session as they were distraught and frightened by where their relationship had landed. They were newly motivated to work on restoring balance in their marriage, which would include better sex. With a humility he had not demonstrated before, Jan admitted that he did not know how to be in his changed marriage with a more assertive wife. He felt that he was losing a grip on who he was and on everything he knew. Jan agreed that he would leave the house if he ever got to the point of wanting to force sex again. Zofia also agreed that she could and would leave the house if tensions escalated. But Zofia responded with compassion to Jan's despair. Instead of focusing on getting an apology, Zofia asked for Jan to change, to be more sensitive to her needs, and to be more caring both sexually and relationally. She wanted help with household tasks, she wanted to know more about their finances, and she wanted sex to be something that was optional, not obligatory.

The decision to work with Jan and Zofia on their sexual relationship and then on other aspects of their relationship dynamic, including Jan's ability to manage his emotions without relying on sex, was a very deliberate choice. In fact, this couple addressed many of their relationship inequities by first addressing them in their sexual relationship. This is not the preferred pathway for every case of relationship distress. However, it can be an option because the reverse (first working on the relationship and then on sex, or assuming that sex will automatically improve) is also not the best pathway for every case that presents for couples therapy.

Jan and Zofia were ready to work on their sexual relationship as a pathway toward repairing their marriage. They did not have the skills to do this themselves; they needed help, as do many couples when their relationships change as a result of trauma, or as a result of the therapy process itself. Sometimes couples need guardrails, and therapists need to be ready to provide them in the form of structure and boundaries and, as in Jan and Zofia's case, plans to stay safe. With the new ceasefire in place, Jan and Zofia needed a structured approach to a more lasting reconciliation. This is where exercises can be helpful.

Prescribing Sexual Exercises

Reading the literature on sex therapy, one might be forgiven for thinking that all sex therapists are exercise fanatics—prescribing sexual homework or exercises so their patients might have more and better sex. While it is true that exercises or homework are often part of the process, there is nothing magical or compulsory about them. When necessary, sex therapists simply help couples approach aspects of their sexual relationship that they might otherwise avoid so they have the opportunity to experience their sexuality in more pleasurable ways.

Sensate focus is the most well-known of the sex therapy techniques developed by Masters and Johnson (1970). Sensate focus refers to a series of invariant exercises that progress from nongenital to genital stimulation through predetermined stages. The preliminary aim of sensate focus is to turn attention toward the sensual aspects of touch (pressure and temperature) and away from judgmental or anxious thoughts that interfere with sexual pleasure (Does my partner like this? Am I getting an erection?). Subsequent phases of sensate focus allow for communication and the sharing of information about partners' experiences.

Masters and Johnson (1970) sought to reduce performance anxiety by creating a series of exercises focusing first on touching for one's own interest rather than the pressured situation of trying to sexually arouse another person. But sexual problems are not just manifestations of performance anxiety gone awry. What some lament as a misuse of sensate focus (e.g., instructions to provide pleasure, to communicate, to arouse; Weiner & Avery-Clark, 2014) may in fact be the natural development or broadened application of a helpful set of exercises. The interested reader can refer to an illustrated manual describing sensate focus as Masters and Johnson intended (Weiner & Avery-Clark, 2017), and Linda Weiner's instructions for the first phase of sensate focus can be found in Appendix C. Once familiarized with the traditional method of sensate focus, I do encourage creative adaptations suitable for the couple currently in treatment.

Jan and Zofia were motivated to find new ways to relate to one another, but they did not know how to go about this. When considering asking the couple to do something (e.g., prescribing an exercise), there are two key questions that need to be answered: (a) What is the goal? and (b) Does the couple need the guidance of a therapist? For Jan and Zofia, the answer to the second question was yes. They were struggling, and Jan was clearly not coping well. The goal of asking the couple to do something together at home may be as basic as wanting to understand more about how they interact with each other. Do they complete the assignment? Is one person more eager or reluctant? Can they communicate with each other? Are they ready to be sensual, if not sexual, with each other? For Jan and Zofia, the overall goal of treatment was to improve their relationship. The goal of the sexual exercises was to help Jan become a more sensitive lover and to help Zofia be more assertive regarding her own needs and desires. So their first exercise involved interrupting the sex that was tediously focused principally on Jan's pleasure and on intercourse.

A moratorium on intercourse is one way to interrupt a tedious routine. If the goal is not to have intercourse, the questions that face the couple become "What and why are we doing anything?" There is no end point, except perhaps pleasure. Finally, pleasure becomes the focus, and routines are interrupted. So for the next few weeks, if and when they had sex, they agreed not to have intercourse. I told Jan that it was his responsibility to maintain this boundary, even if Zofia begged for intercourse (a prospect that brought some laughter to them both). Jan, not Zofia, was to hold the line. This stipulation was put in place to build trust that Jan could control his sexual urges and also to give Zofia the space to experience desire, something she could not do if she always had to worry about having, or not having, sex.

I suggested that they take turns giving each other sexual pleasure, rather than mutually and simultaneously engaging with one another. The purpose was that, at least for a time, Jan would have to focus on Zofia's pleasure instead of his own. And Zofia would likewise have to focus on her pleasure. She would need to communicate to Jan what she liked so that he could do more of it.

So, they left the session with a homework assignment to focus on taking turns giving each other pleasure (with Jan to pleasure Zofia first—to correct for years of her pleasure being an afterthought). Jan asked if they were "allowed" or "supposed to" have orgasms. I said that their responses would be in reaction to whatever they were feeling in the moment. The goal was not orgasm, although if that happened it was fine, and if it did not, that was fine too. The purpose was to have fun, to explore what felt good, and to communicate. I set a time limit of 20 minutes of pleasuring before they switched to the other person, wanting there to be some accountability toward equal time and opportunity for pleasure. Twenty minutes of touching, kissing, and caressing another person is actually a fair bit of time and requires some focus and creativity.

Developing exercises is a creative and collaborative process with couples in therapy. Initially, I often need to be more directive, with the couple agreeing to or modifying my suggestions. As therapy progresses, I may take a back seat and let the couple discuss what they would like their assignment to be for the next few weeks. And then hopefully, I become irrelevant to that process.

Although the exercises for Jan and Zofia were focused on sex, they also targeted the problematic and underlying relationship dynamics. The sexual exercises were creating an equitable balance within the relationship; they were helping the couple integrate Zofia's needs, wants, desires, and pleasure into the relationship, and they were restoring Jan's sense of being valued and cared for by being pleasured and by becoming a more capable, competent, and responsible lover for his wife.

A word of advice: If you ask couples to do an exercise at home, follow up in the next session, especially if the exercise involves abstinence. One couple told me that their therapist advised them not to have sex for a while. Three months later they had not discussed sex in their therapy, and their relationship was on the brink. When finally one of them asked about sex, the (now former) therapist had no recollection of having ever given that advice.

Exercises Are Not Always Necessary

Jan and Zofia needed specific exercises and guidance, but sometimes I am awed by the ability of my patients to come up with creative ways to address their problems without my "brilliant" exercises. Sometimes it is enough to allow people the time and space to reflect on their sexual dynamics and to work through their issues at their own pace. I will share two stories of such couples with you.

An older African American couple, Albert and Rose, were encountering difficulties adjusting to Albert's retirement from a busy and demanding career. They stopped having sex because their relationship was faltering. Rose found herself frequently annoyed with Albert for being underfoot, and she was short-tempered and cross with him often. Albert did not respond verbally to her annoyance; instead, he withdrew into silence, which only further troubled her. In one session, Rose accused Albert of not even knowing his own feelings. She suggested that perhaps they use a feelings wheel or chart similar to those she had used in her days as an elementary school teacher. Albert exploded: "I know what my feelings are, and I don't need children's toys to help me! God damn it, Rose, I had to shut my mouth for years at work, and now it's happening at home!" I knew that Albert was referencing the racial discrimination he had experienced and had described in an earlier session. Mistaken for a janitor or a construction worker unless he was impeccably dressed, even on a worksite, this talented architect had borne it all with silence and a smile. Rose was angry. She felt she did not deserve his anger and told him so. She had been his emotional support all those years, and this was the thanks she got? She, too, had experienced racism and sexism! This heated argument occurred at the end of the session, and I worried, as they both stormed out of the office, that I had not had time to help them reach a better resolution.

The next week, they arrived smiling and happy. Albert had driven straight to a bookstore following the session and picked up an anthology of poetry. Over the next few days, he rewrote several poems in order to express his intimate feelings to Rose. "I know how I feel, and I feel a lot of other things besides anger," Albert said in the session. "But I do find the words to express those feelings often elude me. So now I have Tennyson, Byron, Yeats, and others to help me out." Rose was beaming. Now she did not need to guess about his feelings. Communication improved, and sex resumed. I never would have come up with such an elegant solution.

The other humbling experience was one involving a newly married couple, Brittany and Sean. They had waited until marriage to do much of anything sexually, ostensibly for religious reasons. But in addition to their religion, both were anxious about sex. Brittany had been shamed about her body and her sexuality by her zealously religious stepmother. She had trouble even subtly signaling to Sean that she was interested in sex. Sean had been abused as a child by a high school coach, and he was anxious that he would become an abuser. He had to be certain that Brittany wanted sex before he could initiate. You see the problem.

In one session, Brittany was lamenting that it had been weeks since Sean had "come after me." "Wait," I said. "Is this what you call initiating sex?" They both agreed that it was. "You have to find different words," I said. "'Coming after you' seems rather aggressive, especially given Sean's concerns." They left the session puzzled about what to do. But the next week they returned quite pleased with themselves and reported that they had had sex twice (a record for them). "What happened?" I asked. They were discussing the session over coffee when Brittany noticed how much sugar Sean was spooning into his cup. "You sure like sugar," she said. And voila! They had it. They decided that either of them could ask the other if they wanted sugar when they were interested in sex. And to add icing to the proverbial cake (to continue the sugar metaphor), one night Brittany left a packet of sugar on Sean's pillow, which was accepted and understood as the sexual invitation it was. Again, I never would have come up with such a sweet solution.

SUMMARY

Couples therapy differs in many ways from individual therapy, requiring that therapists hold multiple perspectives at the same time while balancing the often-competing needs of the individuals in the couple. When discussing sexual issues with a couple, there is a need for well-defined and well-communicated boundaries, as therapists will differ on the limits of confidentiality and the keeping of secrets within the therapeutic relationship. But when a relationship is problematic, couples therapy is often the ideal place to work. A couple's sexual relationship provides an intimate reflection of the larger relational dynamics. And working on improving a couple's sexual relationship can be a way of not just improving sex but also addressing other problematic dynamics in the relationship. A couple's sexual relationship is especially vulnerable during times of transition, and sexual difficulties may mirror the difficulties that the couple is experiencing as they attempt to adjust to a new reality. It is always important to talk about the timeline for the development of sexual problems and to ask specifically when the couple first noticed that "something was wrong." Sometimes, addressing sexual issues will entail homework exercises, but sometimes it will not. Homework, as with other interventions, will depend on what the couple needs.

9 PROBLEMATIC PORNOGRAPHY

In 1964, when United States Supreme Court Justice Potter Stewart was asked to define pornography, he famously responded, "I know it when I see it" (as cited in Gewirtz, 1996, p. 1023). Since then, the task of defining pornography has not gotten any easier.

Pornography continues to defy simple definitions and simplistic assertions of whether it is harmful or beneficial. Many people enjoy watching pornography, which I will define rather generally as sexually explicit materials designed to sexually arouse. The negative connotation assigned to the words "porn" or "pornography" has greatly lessened over the years, as pornography use has become much more common. While many people watch porn alone, some couples enjoy viewing pornography together. But sometimes pornography is a point of contention in a relationship, and couple therapists often find themselves in the uncomfortable position of facilitating a discussion about porn. It is an uncomfortable position because therapists may sometimes bring to the discussion their own assumptions and reactions to pornography. It is also uncomfortable because patients are often defensive, ashamed, or confused by their own or their partner's use of porn. This chapter explores pornography use in a distressed couple who were also confronting fears of

https://doi.org/10.1037/0000483-010
Talking About Sex in Psychotherapy: A Guide for Every Therapist, by K. S. K. Hall

infertility and ambivalence about parenthood. As this case illustrates, sex was not just a problem in the relationship; it was also a therapeutic technique, a way to help the couple improve their intimacy and communication.

NILA AND THEO

Nila and Theo were uncomfortable in my office. Nila sat in the armchair, and Theo perched on the couch, with the emptiness of the seat next to him quite obvious. Theo started by saying that he was here to help Nila heal from his betrayal: "I hurt Nila very badly, and I want to make it up to her. I want her to trust me again." Nila said she hoped for the same, for healing and for trust to be rebuilt, but she was doubtful it could happen.

"What happened to damage the trust between you?" I asked, to neither of them in particular, waiting to see who would answer. Theo swallowed hard, looked at Nila, then at me. They had obviously agreed that he should talk.

> I have a sex addiction. I'm in recovery. I've been sober for about 3 months now. But before I started going to a group for porn addicts, I was pretty much out of control. [He glances at Nila and corrects himself.] No, I was out of control. I used porn, a lot. Excessively. And I had an affair. It wasn't love. It was an obsession. But it's over now.

Theo and Nila had been married for almost 3 years when they came to see me. Theo was 35, and Nila was 31 years old. Theo came from a large and boisterous family. He was the middle of five children surrounded on both sides by professionally and financially successful siblings. He was looking forward to becoming equally successful and then having a family of his own one day. Nila shared the dream of a family, and to her that meant having a house full of children. Nila was an only child and grew up wishing for siblings. Her family moved a lot during her childhood, so she did not have a consistent friendship group or best friend. She wanted her children never to feel the loneliness she had experienced. Nila relied on Theo to be her best friend, her husband, her emotional support, and the future father of her children.

Nila and Theo met online, and even though they lived almost 500 miles apart, they enjoyed talking with one another, and soon Theo was flying to see Nila about every 2 months. After a year of long-distance dating, they married, and Nila moved to New Jersey, setting up a home in the condo that Theo owned. Theo had a well-paying job and was happy to support the couple while Nila looked for work. They had both agreed that they would work, save to buy a bigger home, and then start a family. In the meantime,

Theo was looking forward to enjoying life as a dual-income, no-kids couple. But Nila was having trouble finding a job that suited her, and after a year of living with Theo, she was still not employed. Nila complained that she felt lonely and that Theo worked such long hours (to make more money, he said). Nila proposed that they start a family now since she was not working, but Theo was adamant that they needed to save more money and have a bigger home before they had children.

As they sat in my office, now 3 years into their marriage, I could see that Nila was angry with Theo for having an affair, for using porn, for keeping her lonely, for spending money when he was so adamant about saving, and for not being willing to start a family. Theo was sorry.

The couple's stated goals for therapy were to rebuild trust so that intimacy and sex could be restored. In my mind, I was fairly certain that intimacy and sex would need to be improved rather than restored or reinstated. Their failure to work together toward a mutually agreed upon goal (save for a house, have children, or enjoy life as a dual-income couple), their poor communication as evidenced in session, and their agreement that their sex life had only ever been just "fine" or "okay" led me to that conclusion.

As instructed by his addiction group, Theo had given Nila his passwords so that she could access all his devices, and he had installed software to limit his ability to visit adult websites. Nila was able to track Theo's whereabouts at all times, and when she was anxious, she would text him and he would send her a photo of where he was. Nila routinely checked the browsing history on Theo's computer and phone. They were not building trust; they were relying on monitoring tools that reinforced the belief that Theo was not to be trusted. Building trust means taking small, calculated risks, and this couple was not doing that.

Using One Therapist for Both Couples and Individual Therapy: Clarifying Boundaries

Often, when individual therapy is an appropriate complement to couples therapy, couples therapists will refer members of the couple to other therapists to do the individual work. I believe that if boundaries are clear and there is a strong motivation for the couple to stay together, there can be an advantage to having only one therapist for both individual and couples therapy. This approach can be very helpful for couples who have been keeping sexual secrets from each other.

As a first step with Theo and Nila, we agreed that there would need to be a more complete understanding of Theo's porn use and infidelity. This would best be done in individual sessions in order to help Theo be more honest in his disclosures. Theo needed to understand what had caused him to have an affair and to use porn daily, and then he could share his insights with Nila. Simply saying he had an addiction would keep them locked into a position of mistrust and monitoring. An important question to answer was this: To what degree was Theo's sexual acting out a function of an unhealthy relationship dynamic, or to what extent was it a preexisting or separate behavior that he brought into the relationship?

Nila needed therapy to process the hurt and anguish she felt as a result of Theo's betrayal. She would be best able to explore her own issues in therapy away from Theo, to whom she related solely as an injured party. Nila needed to look at her own functioning in the marriage beyond being a victim. So I made the suggestion, and they agreed, to have regularly scheduled individual sessions in addition to biweekly couples therapy. Individual sessions would be confidential. If they decided to end couples therapy or to end their marriage, I would not be available to serve either of them as their individual therapist, given that I was their couples therapist. With boundaries clearly spelled out, we proceeded.

Sex Addiction or Compulsion?

What Theo meant when he said that he had a sex addiction is that he found himself spending more and more of his time and mental energy on porn sites. He tried to control himself; he tried to use willpower to stop, but he was unable to do so. When he became frightened that he was spiraling out of control, Theo told Nila about his addiction. That stopped the spiral but ushered in a whole new set of problems.

Nila did not know what to think about Theo's addiction. "Was it just an excuse for bad behavior, or could he really have an addiction, a problem out of his control, like alcoholism?" Nila's uncertainty mirrors the confusion that many clinicians experience when confronted with patients who self-diagnose as having sex addiction. While the term may have descriptive power (strong urges that feel uncontrollable, resulting in repetitive sexual behavior that has negative impacts), it does not help uncover or explain the complexity of such dysregulated sex or the psychology of the person behind the sexual behavior.

There is no formally recognized diagnosis of sex addiction in the *DSM-5*. The current edition of the *DSM* as well as previous editions of the diagnostic manual have declined to include a category of sexual addiction or hypersexuality, citing insufficient evidence (American Psychiatric Association,

2022). Attempts to find a chemical substrate of sex addiction (e.g., an addiction to the release of opiate-like chemicals in the brain during sex) have failed. Sex may be similar to other behaviors that, at a high frequency, share many of the same components of chemical addictions but are better conceptualized as behavioral addictions (e.g., gambling, video gaming; Bőthe, Nagy, et al., 2024; Griffiths, 2005).

Eschewing the addiction conundrum, the latest edition of the *International Statistical Classification of Diseases and Related Health Problems* (11th ed.; *ICD-11*; World Health Organization, 2019) has included a new diagnosis of compulsive sexual behavior disorder (CSBD). According to the *ICD-11*, CSBD is "characterized by a persistent pattern of failure to control intense, repetitive sexual impulses or urges, resulting in repetitive sexual behaviour over an extended period (e.g., 6 months or more) that causes marked distress or impairment in personal, family, social, educational, occupational or other important areas of functioning" (Kraus et al., 2018, p. 109). The stipulation of a duration of 6 months or more, along with the criteria of distress and/or impairment, is to avoid pathologizing sexual behavior that is otherwise transitory or is problematic only in that it violates a person's moral code. Problematic pornography use (PPU) is the most common behavioral manifestation of CSBD (Bőthe, Vaillancourt-Morel, et al., 2024). Throughout this chapter, I use PPU rather than pornography addiction or sex addiction, unless that is the terminology of the patient.

Problematic or Nonproblematic Pornography Use?

Viewing and masturbating to pornography is quite common in the general population; large-scale and nationally representative surveys show that 70% to 94% of adults and 42% to 98% of adolescents report using pornography (Bőthe, Nagy, et al., 2024). Population estimates of the prevalence of PPU are, of course, much lower at 3.2% to 16.6%, with the highest levels being reported by men and gender-diverse individuals (i.e., individuals who do not identify as exclusively male or exclusively female) as well as people from more conservative cultures.

Many couples watch porn together, often with the stated intention of spicing up their sex lives. In general, greater relationship and sexual satisfaction as well as better sexual communication have been reported for heterosexual couples who watch porn together (Huntington et al., 2021). This rosy picture is moderated by the need to consider the context in which pornography viewing happens. For couples who share sexual values and desires, watching porn together is related to increased sexual satisfaction and intimacy. But remember: Correlation is not causation. Being bullied or coerced into watching pornography in the context of an abusive relationship will not improve the relationship and will likely worsen it. The aggressiveness that is often depicted in pornography may reinforce already-abusive behavior and may even provide a model for engaging in sexually coercive, aggressive, or demeaning activities. Context matters. Therapists should exercise caution before suggesting that couples view porn together in order to increase desire and excitement. A better strategy is to help couples navigate their independently made decision to view porn together: How will they choose what to watch? Who has veto power? When will they watch? How often? Can they also watch on their own? Can they change their minds and not watch porn?

Men, like Theo, who are in relationships but watch pornography on their own, may watch content that they would not want to share with their partner (the aggressive and sadistic nature of the pornography Theo later acknowledged watching would fit into this category). Men's solo pornography watching is related to decreased relationship satisfaction and higher levels of distress in their partners (Bőthe et al., 2018; Bőthe, Nagy, et al., 2024; Bőthe, Vaillancourt-Morel, et al., 2024). The directionality of this relationship is not obvious from this correlation; many men may watch pornography to compensate for an unsatisfying relationship, while others will create distance and dissatisfaction in the relationship because of their preference for solo porn use. Wegmann et al. (2025) found that both positive reinforcement (sexual gratification) and negative reinforcement (compensation or relief from negative mood states) were important to the development and maintenance of PPU. Whatever the initial motivation for watching pornography, the gratification from viewing pornography stays high even when the viewer is facing real or potential negative consequences for viewing it. Theo's porn use may have distracted him from attending to aspects of the relationship he found unsatisfying, or he may have been creating distance and contributing to Nila's loneliness by virtue of his nightly retreats into his study.

The situation is different for women. Partnered women who watch pornography on their own tend to watch porn that is congruent with their relationship values. They use pornography as a way to explore their own sexuality, perhaps empowering them to ask for their (possibly newly discovered) sexual needs to be met in partnered activity and facilitating their sexual responsiveness (Huntington et al., 2021; Vaillancourt-Morel et al., 2021). To extrapolate these findings to same-sex and gender-diverse couples, the message to all couples may be best summarized thus: Viewing pornography whose content is congruent with relationship values may enhance a relationship, while viewing pornography that is incongruent will likely result in distress and damage to an existing relationship.

ASSESSING PORNOGRAPHY USE

In crafting the diagnosis of CSBD for the *ICD-11*, the authors cautioned clinicians to carefully evaluate individuals who self-diagnose a sex or porn addiction, as Theo did (Kraus et al., 2018). Recent research is helpful in knowing which factors to look for when patients report having a porn addiction such that moral incongruence is differentiated from PPU. Moral incongruence, the feeling that one's behavior and one's values are misaligned, is frequently associated with internet pornography use (Grubbs et al., 2022) but is not sufficient for a diagnosis of CSBD.

Based on my review of the literature and my clinical experience, I consider five factors when exploring a patient's pornography use. None of these factors in isolation determines PPU, and clinical judgment is essential.

Salience

The importance of pornography to a particular patient can be partly deduced by asking about the frequency of use and the length of time spent viewing pornography. While the frequency of pornography use is the strongest predictor of problematic use, on its own it is not highly informative. High-frequency pornography use may be due to strong sexual desire, for example. Other factors, as listed in this section, must be considered in determining whether pornography use is problematic (Bőthe, Vaillancourt-Morel, et al., 2024).

Motivation

Certain motivations for viewing pornography are associated with problematic use, while others are not. Viewing porn for sexual pleasure or to increase sexual excitement is the number one reason that most people view pornography. But it is not the only reason, and it is not naive to ask, "What motivates you to watch porn?" Or more simply put, "Why do you watch porn?" Sometimes viewing pornography allows the viewer to engage in fantasy and thus experience imaginary scenarios that would be hard to create in real life. Sexual curiosity (to gain new ideas for sexual engagement) is a motivation for viewing pornography that resonates with women. The motivation for self-exploration, a desire that is expressed by women, gender-diverse individuals, and members of sexual minorities, is a desire to explore what feels good and what does not; it is about exploring one's sense of pleasure rather than exploring ideas about what one might do sexually (the sexual curiosity motivation; Koós et al., 2024). Gay and bisexual men report that they use pornography for inspiration in terms of what sexual activities they might like to engage in with a partner (Demant et al., 2024). Transpersons describe using pornography to imagine having a different body and to imagine possibilities. They also note that seeing transpeople being objectified and fetishized in porn is a negative experience (Pavanello Decaro et al., 2023).

Problematic motivations for viewing pornography include boredom avoidance, emotional suppression, stress reduction, and compensating for a lack of sexual satisfaction in partnered activity. These problematic motivations are associated with poor relationship adjustment as well as self- and partner distress (Bőthe, Vaillancourt-Morel, et al., 2024). Pornography, when used to avoid or cope with negative feelings, can contribute to anxiety, depression, sexual problems, and emotional dysregulation, which in turn can lead to or worsen PPU (Varod et al., 2024). So, after inquiring in general about motivations for viewing pornography, follow-up questions are helpful. For example, at one point I asked Theo, "Do you ever watch porn to avoid feeling angry or disappointed with Nila?" (Theo's answer: Yes. A lot.)

Although most people masturbate while watching porn, at least some of the time, it is important to note that masturbation and orgasm do not necessarily occur with every encounter with pornography. If pornography is not used for sexual gratification, then other motivations become more important to uncover.

Conflict

PPU is also associated with interpersonal conflict, relationship distress, and avoidance of the partner, partnered sex, or other intimacy (Bőthe et al., 2022). Areas of conflict or conflict avoidance should be assessed. PPU is also associated with internal conflict, including sexual shame as well as the experience of moral incongruence. When inquiring about patients' feelings and thoughts before and after pornography use, many patients report feeling ashamed, embarrassed, or guilty. To determine whether these feelings of guilt are solely or primarily about the morality of pornography, it is helpful to ask what the patient thinks about pornography in a general sense, what they believe others would think of pornography or what others would think if they knew the patient was viewing pornography, and what their religious education (if any) has taught them about pornography. Moral incongruence is a sufficient reason for shame but not a necessary one. Clinicians need to be sensitive to the possibility that guilt and shame may be triggered by other memories and experiences from the patient's personal history, including exposure to pornography in the context of sexual abuse.

Escalation

PPU is often marked by an escalation of use over time in terms of the frequency of use or the sexual content portrayed. Greater frequency or increasingly graphic content is sometimes required to achieve the same level of sexual gratification that was once previously experienced (Bőthe, Nagy, et al., 2024). Asking for a timeline and inquiring about the frequency of use and the content of porn across that timeline can ascertain whether the pornography use is escalating.

Control

PPU is marked by unsuccessful attempts to stop or reduce pornography use. There is a shift toward negative mood states when watching pornography is not possible (Bőthe, Nagy, et al., 2024). In addition to asking about the number of times the patient tried to stop watching porn, it is also important to understand the lengths they went to in their efforts to stop (e.g., blocks on computer vs. willpower). It is also helpful to know what happened that brought them back to viewing pornography (events, thoughts, mood states).

ASSESSMENT SCALES

There are several scales that may further guide assessment of whether a patient's use of pornography is problematic. The Problematic Pornography Consumption Scale (PPCS; Bőthe et al., 2018), along with its briefer version, the PPCS-6 (Bőthe et al., 2021), and the Brief Pornography Screen (BPS; Kraus et al., 2020) have excellent psychometric properties. Clinicians may want to use these scales to assess or screen for PPU, and then follow up with their own questions, or they may choose to incorporate the questions into the clinical interview. The brief screening tools will help identify who might be at risk for PPU, while the PPCS will be more helpful in identifying existing problematic use. The Pornography Use Motivations Scale (PUMS) and its briefer version, PUMS-8, are similarly helpful in framing questions or for use in determining problematic motivations for pornography use (Koós et al., 2024).

THEO'S USE OF PORN

Theo described an evening ritual of watching porn. After finishing dinner, he would tell Nila that he had some work to do. He would go into his home office and watch porn. He spent a great deal of time picking out what he liked. Then after viewing and masturbating, he would open an Excel spreadsheet in which he rated the porn based on how arousing it was, the attractiveness of the actors, and the quality of the production. He was not sure why he kept the spreadsheet because he never went back to view porn he had already seen. However, Theo felt that perhaps it helped him "wind down" so he could join Nila for the remainder of the evening (which usually was not a long time). Although there were plenty of free pornography websites, Theo began paying subscription fees, hoping for better-quality porn (according to his three measures of arousal, attractiveness, and production value). He paid for subscriptions so that he would not be distracted by advertisements, and he was drawn in by the promise of especially sadistic content. Surprisingly, Theo was not disturbed by the sadistic content of the porn he preferred: "I know it's not real, and I know for certain that I have no interest in inflicting harm on anyone. It's just, it's like watching a sexy horror movie and all your senses are on high alert." What Theo felt guilty about was taking time away from Nila and spending money from their joint savings account on something that Nila would surely object to. Theo felt guilty that he preferred watching porn to having sex with Nila, and he acknowledged that the quality and frequency of their mutual sexual encounters had suffered, as had the emotional intimacy in his marriage.

As I describe my questions for Theo, you will note that they share a great deal of similarity with the questions on these screening questionnaires. For example, the BPS is a five-item inventory, and one of the items is "You find yourself using pornography more than you want to," with respondents choosing between three options: never, occasionally, and very often. Theo had already told me that pornography was a problem when he shared that he had a porn addiction. I asked Theo the following questions: "So, you use porn more than you'd like to?" (Theo nods in agreement.) "How often do you use it?" (Theo indicates daily and sometimes twice-daily use for about an hour each time.) "How often do you think would be a healthy amount of porn to use?" (Here, Theo says that no amount of porn is okay for him, given his addiction, but when asked about pornography use in a broader context, he said that he did not see anything wrong with it for people [unlike himself] who could handle it.) "When did you start viewing porn?" (Theo says around 14 years of age, when he got a laptop and had the privacy to view porn.) "When did you start to think you had a problem with porn, whether or not you identified it as an addiction?" (Theo said he started to wonder when he noticed that he was avoiding sex with Nila in order to masturbate to porn.)

The PPCS asks respondents to indicate the frequency of a behavior or an emotional reaction on a 7-point scale from 1 = never to 7 = all the time. One of the items is "I became agitated when I was unable to watch porn." If I had administered the PPCS to Theo, my guess is he would have indicated a 6 or a 7 based on the past 6 months (which is the time frame of interest for all three scales). Instead, I asked Theo the following:

ME: Can you remember a time when you couldn't watch porn for some reason?

THEO: I could always figure out a way to watch porn. But there were times I tried not to, on purpose. I tried to stop. One time, I decided to go for a walk instead. There's this park across the street with a walking path; it's about a quarter-mile loop around a nice pond. I walked around it 20 times—that's 5 miles! My feet were killing me because I was still wearing my work clothes, so I still had my work shoes on. And still, I came home and watched porn.

ME: That is a lot of walking in hard-soled shoes. Apart from foot pain, what were you feeling?

THEO: Jittery, nervous, upset, all the above. And I was definitely upset about being upset about not watching porn. I just kept thinking of what a pathetic human being I am.

ME: Have you tried other strategies to avoid watching porn?

THEO: Oh, sure. Sheer willpower—doesn't work. Distraction, doing something else like exercising—doesn't work, or drinking, trading one vice for another—kind of my methadone maintenance plan for porn. Doesn't work. You know that's why I had the affair, right? So I would stop watching porn. I thought if maybe I could do some of the things I saw in the videos, I'd get it out of my system. It didn't work either.

By the time Theo and Nila came to see me, Theo's use of porn was devoid of pleasure. It was a nightly ritual complete with strategies for choosing the video and for rating the experience afterward. Theo was using pornography to suppress the anger and disappointment he felt toward Nila, and he was using pornography to make up for the unsatisfying sex he was having with

Nila (Bőthe, Nagy, et al., 2024). His use of pornography, however, was making all of this worse.

THEO'S INDIVIDUAL THERAPY

Theo appreciated the opportunity to talk about and explore his feelings about his marriage and his relationship with Nila. He was a responsible man. A great many expectations hung on his shoulders that were not dissimilar to those placed on his siblings, but Theo worried because his sisters and brothers were more successful than he was. He relied on the outward trappings of success to feel some equality with them. Hence, he wanted a bigger house, and he wanted a wife who had a professional job and earned good money. He wanted to have a few years before having children when he and Nila could afford nice vacations and dinners out. He was very disappointed when Nila turned down jobs, saying they were not good enough. He did not know how to talk to her about his concerns because she would ask him, "But you don't want me to take a job that is beneath me? I would be so unhappy." When Nila approached the subject of starting a family, Theo was in despair. It seemed that nothing about this marriage was working out according to his hopes. Money was tight; they could not afford vacations or dinners out. The condo was small and not suitable for a family. His wife did not work, and worse, she did not really seem to do anything all day: no volunteer work, no friends, minimal housework, and plenty of complaining when he came home. When he tried to talk to her, Nila would cry, "I gave up everything to come here and be with you. And now you blame me that I can't find a good job, that I have no friends, and that I have nothing to do all day!"

Theo is a first-generation East Asian American. His parents had an arranged marriage and moved to the United States from India shortly after their wedding. He admired them for their courage and professional success. Theo wanted his parents to think of him as successful as well, so he could not confide in them or any other family members about his unhappiness. He knew that divorce was the worst of all options in the eyes of his parents. So, Theo began watching porn more frequently, and then he began watching porn depicting women in servile roles, having to service men, from cleaning their shoes to performing fellatio. He watched videos in which women were gagged and beaten. After he masturbated and ejaculated, Theo would feel very guilty and would tell himself to try to be kinder to Nila. He thought that perhaps the pornography was helpful in this way (motivating him to kindness). However, it was doing the opposite; his viewing of porn was an avoidance of addressing his unhappiness.

Theo described increasing despair about his marriage and his growing apprehension about the porn he was viewing. He thought that if he could act out some of the scenes he found erotic in the porn, he might get it out of his system. Theo did not recognize this as a justification for engaging in desired behavior about which he felt conflicted. He described how he initiated an affair with a coworker who he knew had a crush on him. He told me that he was relieved to discover that he did not really enjoy acting out the fantasies of domination and humiliation. Although they role-played rape scenes, Theo found it all too disturbing, so he ended the affair. At least, that was his first description of the affair. He would later reveal in therapy that he was intrigued and aroused by these activities and would have continued, but his affair partner broke it off with him. She told him that she did not like their sexual interactions; they made her feel deeply uncomfortable. She did sexual things she did not want to do in order to show him how much she cared, but it never seemed to matter to Theo. When he told me this, about 8 months into therapy, Theo felt deep shame and was able to see how caught up he was in his own disappointment, anger, and sense of failure. In his myopia, he shut out the experiences of his sexual partners—both his affair partner and Nila. Theo was disgusted with his taste in porn, with his behavior with his affair partner, and with himself.

Theo was able to tell me the truth about his behavior because he could talk about his anger and disappointment and his porn use without being judged. He appreciated the questions that prompted him to explore his thoughts, feelings, and behaviors in more depth and from different vantage points. In other words, therapy helped him be honest with himself.

NILA'S INDIVIDUAL THERAPY

Prior to coming to therapy, Theo told Nila about his porn use and his affair in hopes that this would stop him. It was Nila who insisted he go to a group for porn addicts. In therapy, Nila confessed that she was in shock regarding Theo's disclosures. She had no idea that he was watching porn when he told her he was working. Nila was oblivious to what was going on because she was preoccupied with her own issues in the marriage. She was desperately lonely, and instead of reaching out to Theo, she became convinced that having a baby would solve her unhappiness.

Nila spoke to her mother daily, and she told her everything. Nila told her parents about Theo's affair and his pornography use, and they encouraged her to go to marriage therapy. They liked their son-in-law very much and knew him to be a hardworking and kind man. They also wanted their daughter to be happy, and they could not imagine divorce as a path to happiness. Nila had lived with her parents until she married Theo. She lived at home during her college years and was happy to continue living with her mother and father after her graduation. Nila's parents were also immigrants from India. They, too, had an arranged marriage and had come to the United States as newlyweds. Her father worked for an international trade organization, so the family moved to Dubai, London, Texas, and New York before finally settling in North Carolina. Nila's mother was a stay-at-home parent, and she worried for her daughter's safety in the cities in which they lived. Over time and through their travels, mother and daughter grew very close to each other.

Marriage was not what Nila had imagined. She was lonely. All Theo seemed to care about was her finding a job and making money. He was stressed, and preoccupied and busy all the time. He did not seem to notice how much she missed her parents. If they could not go to fancy restaurants, he did not want to go out at all. He watched every penny she spent and scrutinized the housework she did or did not do. Nila asked if they could move to North Carolina, but the answer was always the same one he gave her when she asked about a vacation, going to dinner, and spending more time together: "When you have a job and we can start saving money. . . ." More than anything, Nila did not want to get a job. She wanted Theo to love her even if she did not work. She wanted Theo to pay attention to her, not to her résumé or her cooking or her housework. With her mother's coaching and encouragement, Nila had a conversation with Theo about starting a family, a conversation he agreed likely happened, but he has no memory of it. This is Nila's memory of the conversation:

NILA: Theo, since I can't find a job and I'm home anyway, let's start our family now.

THEO: This house is too small for us, let alone a baby. When you start working and we can save money to buy a big house, we can start having children. It's just not practical in this house. Right? You agree?

NILA: Well, I'm going to stop taking birth control. If you don't want to have children, then you will have to take care of the birth control.

THEO: Fine. I will.

So, Nila stopped taking her oral contraceptives. Soon she was monitoring her menstrual cycle and trying to decipher her ovulation and fertility window. Then, on her mother's advice, she bought a kit to more closely identify the window in which she was fertile. It was 2 days out of her cycle. Nila, by her own account, became "obsessed" with getting pregnant and was not interested in having sex with Theo except for the days during her fertility window. Nila worried that Theo was avoiding having sex with her as a way to avoid pregnancy. Soon, Nila began to berate Theo and shame him into having sex with her. Theo began to have problems getting an erection, and Nila would cry, "Why can't you just do it? Why can't you be a man?" Nila knew she was acting horribly, but she was so miserable living in a small condo with no friends, no family, a husband who ignored her, and no baby.

INFERTILITY

Nila worried about infertility, given that her mother had had difficulty conceiving and, thus, Nila was an only child. Nila would not have met the criterion for a medical diagnosis of infertility, which is defined as the inability to conceive after a year of unprotected sex (Carson & Kallen, 2021). Although technically Nila had been off birth control for more than a year, she and Theo had not been having intercourse frequently. Still, reading some of the research on infertility and sexuality was helpful to me when working with this couple. Viewing Nila's distress through a lens of infertility was helpful in understanding her often-abusive behavior toward Theo and her contribution to the sexual problems the couple experienced.

Nila said that she allowed herself to believe that Theo really wanted a baby too, and she convinced herself that she needed to be forceful so that Theo would get over "his neurotic need for a bigger house." When Nila was focused on getting pregnant, she abandoned her previous efforts to make sex a time for intimate and pleasurable connection with Theo. When trying to get pregnant, the timing of sex becomes dependent on fertility windows rather than sexual desire. And because the focus is on conception rather than pleasure, fertility-focused sex is characterized by less desire, less foreplay, and less arousal (subjectively experienced and physiologically expressed in lubrication and erection). There are higher rates of sexual dysfunction, with an increase in dysfunction occurring during the sex that occurs in the fertile phase (Leeners et al., 2023). This was clearly the case for Nila and Theo. Nila initiated sex in an aggressive manner. She did not even try to make the sex pleasurable for herself. Instead, she focused on trying to get Theo to be erect and then to have him ejaculate intravaginally. Theo soon experienced erectile dysfunction as well as a lack of desire.

Although Nila and Theo are not typical of couples struggling with infertility, many infertile couples will experience sexual problems. There is a wide variation in the reported prevalence of these problems: In women, they range from 11.3% to 87.5%; for men, the range is 8.9% to 84.9%; and for couples, the range is 15.5% to 52.5% (Leeners et al., 2023). It appears that those individuals and couples who struggle the most and the longest with their infertility status have decreasing sexual satisfaction. Infertility affects approximately 13% of women of reproductive age (Carson & Kallen, 2021). Nila was convinced that she would be one of these women and that fertility would be a long and difficult struggle for her, as it had been for her mother. Theo's ambivalence was just another obstacle for Nila. Nila and Theo's difficult and damaged relationship was not a good starting point for a fertility journey that might also be problematic.

Infertility increases the risk of intimate partner violence, psychologically, physically, sexually, and economically (Wang et al., 2022). This is especially true for individuals and couples whose cultural or familial values stigmatize childlessness and lay blame for the situation on the woman. The risk in these cases is that women will be subject to abuse. But infertility is also associated with an increased risk of sexual coercion, especially toward the male partner, as it was in the relationship between Theo and Nila. Among a sample of infertile heterosexual couples, 37% of men and 12% of women reported being coerced into having sex for conception, which was psychologically distressing and led to poor relationship adjustment (Peterson & Buday, 2020).

Infidelity

Initially, Nila was resistant to looking at her own issues and behavior in the marriage, stating that "it was nothing compared to what he did." She had little empathy for Theo's struggles, his sense of disappointment, and the stress he might have experienced as the sole breadwinner and her emotional and social support when she moved in. And she had absolutely no empathy for how her verbally abusive and coercive behavior during sex might have affected him. To be clear, I was never trying to have Nila accept responsibility for Theo's affair or his pornography use; rather, I was encouraging her to accept responsibility for her own emotions and behaviors.

One very key session involved an exploration of something that did not make sense to me. In this case, I was wondering about the fact that Nila seemed rather unperturbed about Theo's affair. She was most distressed by his nightly masturbation to pornography, rather than his affair of several months with a coworker.

ME: So, in all that has happened, the most hurtful thing is that Theo was using porn instead of being with you. What about his affair?

NILA: Men have affairs.

ME: All men?

NILA: My father had an affair; my mother just pretended not to notice. It ended. That's what happened with Theo too. It ended. And also, what I heard in our last couples session was really helpful to me.

ME: What was that?

NILA: When Theo admitted that he hadn't broken off the affair, that it was her. And that she told him it was because he wasn't treating her nicely. And I thought, "Wow. I wish I could do that"—not break up with Theo but stand up for myself like that.

ME: That's interesting.

NILA: You know, I was really angry at Theo for a long time. I really felt that he didn't treat me very well when I moved here. I still think that's true, but I also understand him a bit more, and I also hold myself a bit to blame. I never told him that sex was . . . I don't know how to say this. Sometimes there was not a lot of feeling in it, you know? Like it was mechanical. No tenderness. And then kind of trying to trick him into getting pregnant—that's not great, right?

ME: No, that's not great.

NILA: My mother really just sees my side, and she wants me to have what I want. But maybe that wasn't the best advice.

ME: Standing up for yourself and still being in a loving relationship—a skill to learn with your parents and with Theo.

NILA: I know. I knew it wasn't the best idea. But I wanted to believe that it was okay. This is so confusing. Isn't therapy supposed to bring clarity?

ME: (*smiling*) Who told you that?

NILA: (*laughing*) Stop it! It was not my mother. I just heard it somewhere.

ME: Relationships are complex, and perhaps that's the clarity you are getting now.

As we discussed her lack of jealousy about the affair, I asked Nila if she ever felt jealous of anyone. She told me that she felt extremely jealous on one occasion. She and Theo were visiting friends who had just gotten a new puppy. Theo was playing with the puppy, and Nila saw him being loving and playful and happy, which filled her with a rage of jealousy. "Why isn't he like that with me?" She never told anyone about this, not even her mother, because it felt stupid. However, in our next couples therapy session, Nila shared the story of the puppy with Theo and told him that she wanted to experience that side of him. He acknowledged that he is not often so open and vulnerable. He was pleased that Nila had seen that in him that day: "Maybe I wasn't always invisible to her." Neither of them made the connection to the vision of Theo as a father to a child, so I did not either.

A SEX AND COUPLES THERAPY APPROACH TO TREATMENT

Some may wonder why, with so much hurt and anger concerning sexuality, I would choose to work with this couple directly on their sexual relationship. But the question actually supplies the answer. This couple had so much pain about their sexual relationship that it seemed like the ideal place to center our work.

The first step in the process was to build empathy and mutual understanding. It was pointless, not to mention countertherapeutic, to try to decipher what came first, who did what to whom, and when. So, I asked them to try to see the other's point of view, and I used many of the tried-and-true therapy techniques for building empathy, such as having each of them take and argue the other person's point of view. Here is how Nila was able to articulate Theo's viewpoint, even though she had previously been arguing that he had no right to feel any resentment toward her.

NILA: (as Theo) So I thought I was marrying a strong, independent woman, and when you moved in, you started to depend on me for everything. I was supposed to be the breadwinner, the best friend, the romantic date partner, and then a stud! I'm not a robot you can program whenever you have needs. I want you to take care of yourself sometimes, and I want you to take care of me sometimes too.

NILA: (*starting to cry*) I'm a horrible person; I treated you horribly. You must hate me.

THEO: Of course I don't hate you. It's all my fault. I'm the jerk. I'm really sorry.

ME: Theo, can you be Nila for a moment? See if you can express what you believe her point of view is.

THEO: Right, right. Okay. I'm Nila. Umm, Theo, I gave up a lot for you. I had a job I loved and a boss who was really great to me and valued me.

> I have a really great family, and I have always lived with them, and we always had dinner together and talked about our day, and then I didn't have that anymore, and then you stopped having dinner with me and talking to me about your day, and all you would do was talk about money and how we need a big house and about how I need to get a job. Theo, you were basically a big asshole to me. (This made Nila laugh.)

Many of the issues that we worked on in therapy—communication, empathy, and problem solving as a team—were the same ones that we addressed in our work to repair, or rather improve, their sexual relationship. So although I will describe their therapy in what may appear to be a step-by-step progression, we were always working on many levels simultaneously. Working on their sexuality also helped them confront issues that they would otherwise have avoided or talked around in their therapy sessions.

Before encouraging Theo and Nila to engage sexually with each other, I asked them what they needed in order to take risks to trust each other again, to be sexual with each other again. Theo said that he needed to know that Nila was not going to tell her mother about their sex life, and he added other topics that he wanted to keep private as well: contraception and finances. He could not possibly have sex with Nila, Theo explained, if he knew that her mother was going to be told the details. Nila objected to the broad scope of Theo's requests, saying that she relied on her mother for practical advice and emotional support, and to take that away from her before Theo could fill in the gap would feel cruel. I encouraged them to narrow their focus to sex and privacy regarding their sexual relationship. After some discussion, Nila agreed not to talk to her mother about the details of their sex life (she could tell her mother they were or were not having sex, but not more). Theo agreed to be available for conversations with Nila and to work on being a more patient listener and more emotionally supportive (skills we were actively addressing in the therapy sessions).

I next asked them, "What do you feel comfortable doing, in terms of starting to be sexual together again?" Theo thought they should just see what happens, while Nila said she was not even sure she was ready to be sexual. Like many partners, Nila thought that she could not compete in terms of sex appeal, sexual knowledge, and sexual ability with the actresses in the porn videos. I set some boundaries for them in terms of starting to be sexual: going slowly to build desire rather than foster a sense of obligation, and no penetrative activities, given that their contraceptive issues had not yet been resolved. They agreed on getting into bed naked and hugging.

At the start of each new session, I would ask Theo and Nila to discuss their progress, insights, or thoughts about their sensual intimacy (the terminology they used). In this way, they continued to work on problem solving, communication, being vulnerable, and having fun together. When problems arose, I would turn to them and say: "How would you like to handle this? What do you think you should do?" Talking through and planning sexual exercises helped build empathy and improve communication, and it required each of them to think about and articulate their desires.

After many sessions, as Nila began to experience sexual desire for Theo, she also experienced a level of anger she had not previously felt. She wondered how she could be interested in a man who liked porn—and who liked porn in which women were forced into sex. She started to feel anger about his affair and began asking Theo for details of the affair in angry and accusatory tones, reminiscent of her previous shaming communication. (Nila did not know the details of the pornography that Theo watched, just the outline of what he viewed, e.g., scenarios of forced sex. Likewise, she knew little about the details of the affair.)

NILA: I need to know if Theo forced himself upon Olivia. I have a right to know that.

THEO: I have already told you that I didn't, I didn't. But I should have seen that I just wanted sex and she wanted a relationship. I shouldn't have had an affair at all, and I shouldn't have had an affair with Olivia, and I . . . I don't know. I give up.

ME: Nila, what are your concerns?

NILA: I want to know if Theo had anal sex with Olivia. I want to know that. And if he used a condom. I want to know that.

THEO: I don't know what to say; I thought we agreed no details.

NILA: That's very convenient.

ME: Okay, Nila wants to know if she can trust you, Theo. The two of you have made a lot of progress, and my sense is that it's time to revisit trust from this vantage point. You have been sensually intimate, and you have both shared a wish to be sexual. So, if she shares herself with you sexually, can she trust you, Theo?

NILA: That's exactly it.

ME: But Nila, you are reverting to an old shaming pattern of communicating with Theo, and I wonder what's behind that for you?

NILA: I'm sorry, but I need to know if I could get an STI or if Theo wants anal sex, because I don't want those things.

THEO: I got tested. I showed you the results! And I would never force you to do anything you don't want!

ME: How can Nila know that you won't force her?

THEO: She has to trust me?

ME: Nila?

NILA: I'm having a hard time trusting again. I feel really vulnerable. I can't get hurt again.

ME: Nila, what would you do if Theo asked you to have anal sex?

THEO: I wouldn't . . .

ME: Nila, even though Theo says he won't, what would you do if he did ask you?

NILA: I would tell him no.

ME: And if he kept asking?

NILA: I'd get up and leave.

ME: And if he forced you back?

NILA: Oh, he would never do that. No, I can see him badgering me, but that's it.

ME: And if he badgered you, you'd get up and leave.

NILA: Oh, yes.

ME: So, you can trust yourself to set and keep your boundaries, even if Theo tests them. And you seem to trust that Theo will not be physically abusive or aggressive with you.

NILA: Yes, and yes.

ME: So, what do you need to move forward?

NILA: Reassurance that he's not going to hurt me again.

ME: Can you ask him for that?

NILA: Can you promise me that you won't hurt me again?

THEO: I can promise you that I will never knowingly hurt you. I can guarantee it.

ME: That was good communication, Nila—you asked Theo for what you needed, and Theo, you responded very directly and emphatically. But let's keep building this trust, the trust that, Nila, you have in yourself to be more assertive and communicative, and Theo, that you can be more attentive. So, having these goals, what next steps would you like to take sensually or sexually?

NILA: Maybe I could tell Theo what I like?

THEO: I would really like that.

Theo and Nila decided that before they became more sexual, they would try to add some verbal communication to their sensual intimacy. Nila would try being assertive by asking for certain kinds of sensual touch. And Theo would try to listen and check in with Nila regarding how she was feeling and whether he was being responsive to her requests. To be fair, they decided that they would also do the exercise in reverse, with Theo asking for what he would like and with Nila responding. Nila and Theo practiced communication, empathy, and awareness of their own and each other's desire and pleasure first during sensual exercises (no attempts to arouse and no direct stimulation of breasts and genitals); then they were able to apply those skills as they became sexual with each other. It did not take long before they were enjoying sex together. This meant that they needed to address contraception before they had intercourse. After minimal discussion, Nila offered to put a condom on Theo before they had intercourse. She said she had watched an instructional (she clarified that it was not pornographic) video on the topic. She told Theo that she did not ask her mother for advice; she asked her internet browser.

CODA

Theo found the blocks on his phone and computer helpful in ending his reliance on porn. Whenever he felt the urge to look at porn, the knowledge that Nila was still checking his browser history and the awareness of what the consequences would be (her hurt and pain, her lack of respect for him, and the possible end to their marriage) dissuaded him. He was less and less interested in viewing porn and more able to manage his feelings. According to Theo, his interest in sadistic porn was gone. There is, of course, no way to tell, but Theo was much more engaged in his relationship with Nila.

He could see, in retrospect, that he had unilaterally decided that they would delay having children until he felt an equality with his siblings. Now he knew that when to have a baby was a decision they should make together.

Theo and Nila left therapy enjoying life as a married couple (with one income and a tight budget) and having mutually satisfying sex. About a year later, I received a birth announcement heralding the arrival of their daughter, who to my surprise was preceded by a Siberian husky, who was prominently pictured as a big brother on the birth announcement.

The story of Nila and Theo is not unusual in that couples often present with multiple problems, problems that may exceed their ability to cope, as individuals, as a couple, or both. Nila and Theo were each consumed by their own unhappiness and sought a solution that only further damaged trust, intimacy, and sexuality. They were unaware of each other's emotional distress. Focusing on their sexual difficulties was a way to help them become a couple, learn to communicate, and problem-solve their difficulties together, ultimately allowing themselves to be vulnerable and experience pleasure. These are all tasks and goals that couples therapists routinely address. The only difference with Nila and Theo and many of the cases in this book is that sex was not just the problem—it was also the path to the solution.

SUMMARY

"I know it when I see it" is not a very good measure of PPU. PPU is better assessed by the motivation and consequences of pornography use as well as perceived control (or lack thereof) over the frequency of viewing and the content of the pornography. When pornography is used to avoid issues in a relationship or to passive-aggressively express anger, viewing pornography can have a detrimental effect on a couple. "I know it when I see it" is not a good measure of PPU because of its subjectivity. Many couples enjoy watching pornography together to add some spice to their sex life, and many individuals use pornography as a helpful adjunct to masturbation. Sometimes pornography use is problematic because it presents a moral dilemma for the user. Pornography should not be considered a problem solely on the basis of whether we find it morally acceptable. The research cited in this chapter and the scales that have been developed to assess pornography use will be helpful for clinicians navigating this somewhat controversial terrain. The scales and measures will be particularly helpful for clinicians who are predisposed to have a negative view of pornography.

Couples who come to therapy are often struggling with problems in more than one area of their lives together, and having a presenting complaint of

PPU is no exception. Pornography use is sometimes an attempt to remedy other problems and is sometimes a consequence of other difficulties. The case example used in this chapter also touches on issues related to infertility, which can take an additional emotional toll on a couple and on their experience of sexual pleasure. As noted in previous chapters, when problems affect sex, sex can be a good place to focus therapeutic conversations and interventions.

10 CONSENSUAL NONMONOGAMY

"What's so ethical about cheating?" This question was posed to me by Helen, whose husband wanted to unilaterally open their marriage. "What he wants is to cheat without feeling guilty!" Helen was likely not wrong about her husband's motivation. Consensual nonmonogamy, or ethical nonmonogamy as it is also known, is explicitly not cheating. It is called *consensual* because all parties must agree; it is not a unilateral decision one makes in an existing relationship. It is ethical because everyone involved knows about and agrees to the arrangement.

This chapter follows the stories of three previously monogamous couples who explored consensual nonmonogamy when their relationships hit a bump. Their stories illustrate the challenges and the benefits of renegotiating the emotional and sexual boundaries of a relationship.

INTRODUCING THE COUPLES

Keith met Alex while they were both freshmen in college. In fact, they met during the first week of classes. The attraction was instantaneous, and they were inseparable throughout their college years. Keith recalls feeling joy

https://doi.org/10.1037/0000483-011
Talking About Sex in Psychotherapy: A Guide for Every Therapist, by K. S. K. Hall

and relief when he hooked up with Alex. It was his first sexual experience with another person, and when he realized that Alex wanted a relationship, not just sex, he thought, "I've hit the jackpot. I've found my person." Alex did not feel exactly the same. He recalls thinking, "Oh, this is nice, for now." Fast-forward to 5 years after college graduation, and the ink is still drying on their newly signed mortgage papers when Keith discovers Alex having sex with one of their friends. It was at a New Year's Eve party that Keith will not soon forget. "I didn't even want to go to the party," Keith lamented. "But Alex insisted." In the aftermath of this discovery, Alex told Keith that he had been having sex with other men for the entirety of their relationship. He told Keith that he is polyamorous and wants to have an open relationship. Keith is in shock.

Kim and Laura had a rocky start to their relationship, but they were determined to make it work. They got married during the COVID-19 pandemic, despite Kim's extreme dissatisfaction with their sex life. Kim said she loved Laura and was certain that sex would improve. Laura, perhaps swayed by Kim's confidence, was similarly optimistic. I started seeing them just as the lockdowns for the COVID-19 pandemic were easing. They showed up on my computer screen as I did on theirs. Invariably, as we started each session, I had to ask them to adjust the camera angle so that Kim could be fully in the picture. Two years of sporadic therapy later, their rocky relationship was much smoother and Kim was always completely in the picture when our cameras clicked on. Sex was not much better, however. There were so many parts of Laura's body that Kim could not touch and so many restrictions on what they could do sexually. Kim was no longer certain that sex with Laura would improve, but she was certain that she needed to have a better sex life for herself. So now Kim was asking if they could open their relationship. Laura was reluctant.

Anne had her first major depressive episode shortly after the birth of her daughter, and she has struggled with depression ever since. Her daughter is now 24 years old, the same age that Anne was when she gave birth to her. With therapy and medication, Anne no longer suffers from many of the constraints of her depression. She has a job that she finds fulfilling, a few friendships that she enjoys, and a strong emotional connection with her daughter and her husband, Scott. What she does not have is a satisfying sex life. Anne has no interest in sex, and over the years she has felt alternately guilty, resentful, and resigned about it. What she has not felt is sexual desire. First, out of necessity and later out of choice, Scott has had a vibrant solo sex life. He has experimented with his gender identity and with various kink preferences. Scott and Anne wonder if they should try, yet again, to have a sex life with each other, or if they should open their marriage. To be more precise, they are wondering whether their marriage could survive if Scott had other sexual partners. Anne and Scott are equally intrigued by this possibility.

THE APPEAL OF CONSENSUAL NONMONOGAMY

Consensual nonmonogamy (CNM) refers to relationships that vary in terms of sexual and emotional inclusivity/exclusivity. In her book *Polysecure*, therapist Jessica Fern (2020) argues that people who choose CNM do so because they believe they have the ability to meet the needs of more than one partner and that they will thrive by having their needs (sexual and nonsexual) met by more than one person. Nonmonogamy allows them the freedom to grow and develop in ways that they believe would not be possible within a monogamous union. CNM differs from infidelity in that, with CNM, everyone involved is aware of and consents to the relationship structure. CNM is an umbrella term that encompasses many different types of relationship constellations: *Swinging* involves married or partnered people having sex with other people in the same room or location; it is often a shared sexual activity involving watching a partner have sex with someone else, engaging in group sex, or swapping partners with someone else. *Open marriages* are when spouses may have sex with other people, usually within some defined boundaries set by the married couple. *Polyamory* involves multiple sexual and romantic relationships.[1]

Some people who practice CNM do so because it feels like who they really are, in much the same way that people express feelings of identity congruence with other sexual orientations (gay, heterosexual, bisexual, pansexual). This was how Kim felt. She felt that she was most herself, her authentic self, prior to her relationship with Laura, when she had a couple of lovers at the same time, each of whom knew about the other. Some people arrive at a decision to practice CNM because they become aware that they have different sexual (and nonsexual) needs from their partner. Scott's sexual needs went beyond wanting to have more sex than Anne did. He had come to realize that his sexual interests had developed during his years of solo sex in ways that he was sure did not interest Anne. Anne was intrigued by CNM and open to it because it aligned with her social and political views. Anne identified strongly as a feminist, and insofar as CNM could be seen as countering the patriarchal values inherent in monogamy, she supported it

[1]There are other forms of CNM; the interested reader can consult *Polysecure* (Fern, 2020).

(philosophically speaking, not literally, as in having multiple partners herself). Keith believed that committed partners should be everything to each other: friend, confidant, and lover. However, he was willing to consider CNM if the choice was between an open marriage and losing Alex.

KEITH AND ALEX

Keith was distraught when he and Alex showed up for therapy. He said he would do anything to keep their relationship. He was upset, yes, about the secret sex Alex had been having, but he was full of self-recriminations and highly anxious. He said he wanted to work on opening the relationship so that Alex would be happy. He had not known he was holding Alex back from being his authentic self. He wanted to get started on this process right away. Alex was a bit shell-shocked. He had not expected this reaction; rather, he had thought that Keith would end the relationship. "Do you want to end the relationship?" I asked Alex. "Honestly, I don't know."

This was not the time for Keith and Alex to open their relationship. Their relationship was in serious trouble. Keith was in panic mode, and Alex was uncertain. Had Alex purposefully cajoled Keith into coming to the New Year's party so that he would "out himself"? "Honestly, I don't know." Without a strong commitment to each other, opening the relationship did not make sense. There was a strong possibility that this relationship would not last. Keith needed time to process the betrayal of knowing that Alex had had multiple sexual partners over the years they were together. Then he needed to process whether he wanted to have a nonmonogamous relationship, and if so, he would have to give some thought as to what that would look like for him. My questions were these:

- Is Alex really polyamorous, or was he acting out?
- Is Keith's behavior smothering?
- How did Keith not know something was amiss?
- Why was Alex so reckless in terms of having sex at the New Year's party where Keith would likely see?
- Does it have anything to do with the fact that they just bought a house together?

It was interesting that Alex and Keith came to therapy together. They obviously cared a great deal about each other, but they were having trouble having an honest relationship. Over time, this is what we discovered: Alex was terrified of being trapped in a relationship. Growing up in a rural community, he had churchgoing parents who said they loved him but that he should not "practice homosexuality." Every Sunday his mother prayed for him, and his father had periodic check-ins with Alex to make sure he was staying on the right path (celibacy). But despite the reassurances he gave his father, Alex had plenty of sex during his teenage years.

> I knew most of the guys were straight; they likely thought I was too, but we jerked each other off or sucked each other off all the time looking at hetero porn and talking about the girls we'd like to do this to. It felt pretty cool to be fooling my parents, and to be fooling these guys. I got off on it.

Keith's coming-out story was quite different. When Keith told his parents he was gay, they hugged him and said they already knew or were pretty sure. They told him that his happiness was most important, they were glad he told them, it must have been difficult to hold such a secret, and they hoped he would one day find the love of his life as they had. Keith's family also lived in a rural community, and his parents had grown up together and attended the same church. They were childhood sweethearts who married and worked hard for what they had. Keith greatly admired their relationship. He knew that accepting his sexual orientation did not come easily for his parents and that they would suffer from the negative opinions of neighbors and extended family. Nevertheless, they remained staunchly proud of their son. Keith felt so grateful to his parents, and he wanted to deserve their pride, so he worked hard in school, got good grades, did volunteer work, and stayed out of trouble. He did not have sex with anyone until he met Alex. He was waiting, he said, for the love of his life.

In therapy, Alex and Keith shared stories of their lives and discussed their relationship. Keith recognized that he was continuing to try to feel deserving of his parents' pride, to be the gay son they could be proud of. To do anything else made him feel anxious. He thought, in retrospect, that he may have pushed Alex into a relationship and into buying a house before Alex was really ready. Keith thought he might have pushed because he wanted this relationship to be the forever one, and because Alex was a man his parents could feel proud to call a son-in-law.

Alex came to understand that honesty in a relationship was difficult for him. He had never really been honest in his relationships with parents, siblings, friends, or lovers. Deception and sex were intricately tied together for Alex. The sex he had "on the side" was so much more exciting than the sex he had with Keith. It was rebellious, and it made him feel powerful.

Alex and Keith acknowledged that they had a pretty satisfying sexual relationship (even though Alex found the transgressive sex more exciting). They had had only sporadic and somewhat desultory sex with each other since that New Year's Eve discovery. Keith said that he could only be open sexually when he was in a loving relationship. Now that he was unsure about Alex's love, he had lost desire. Alex wondered whether he could enjoy the intimacy of sex with Keith only when he had a secret. Now that he was in therapy, and now that Keith knew about his other sexual experiences, he was having difficulty enjoying sex. Yet he still "did sex"; he felt he owed it to Keith.

At one point in the therapy, I turned to Alex and said:

> I'm confused. You buy a house with Keith, which is a big commitment. Then you ask him to a party where you are pretty sure you will hook up with someone else. And you're pretty sure that Keith will find out, or see you. Which of course he did. So, if you wanted to sabotage the relationship, why did you come to therapy with him, and why have you been working so hard in therapy? Why not just leave?

His answer? "I honestly don't know." I proposed an alternative hypothesis: that Alex wanted to be honest with Keith but could not do it on his own, hence the New Year's Eve party. Keith loved this idea. It would salvage his dream of having found the love of his life, who finally wanted to be an honest man. Alex said, in not so many words, not so fast.

ALEX: I'm not so sure I'm that good a person.

ME: Okay, that's fair. So, why are you working so hard at this relationship now?

ALEX: Because I'm not so sure I'm that bad a person either?

KEITH: You're not a bad person! I really hate it when you say that.

ME: Keith, you might consider that Alex is, as he says, not that good and not that bad.

KEITH: I don't even know what that means.

ME: Alex, can you help out here?

ALEX: I think Dr. Hall means that you need to accept that you love a flawed person.

KEITH: (*looking at me*) Is that right?

ME: I couldn't have said it better.

KEITH: I don't even know how to do that; I mean, I know he's not perfect, but this is confusing.

ME: Well, unfortunately, our time is up for today. Why don't you both think about this, and we can pick it up when we meet next week?

KEITH: Really? Can you at least suggest a book or a podcast or something?

ME: Even if I knew of something, I would rather hear your thoughts and experiences next week. Let this percolate and see what comes up for you.

Over the next several sessions, we processed what it meant for the two of them to know that Alex—and, yes, also Keith—were flawed people. Keith realized that he needed to stop trying to fit Alex into the narrative that he was attached to: that true love leads to happily-ever-after scenarios in which everything is perfect. Alex processed the toll his double life had taken on him, not really knowing who he was because he sometimes could not distinguish truth from his own lies.

The decision to open the relationship came after a year of therapy, and it came from Keith: "I think it's time to open the relationship." This pronouncement was a bit shocking to Alex, but not to me. This was not the rush to save his relationship as the motivation to open the relationship had been when we first met. Keith was not suggesting CNM to appease Alex; Keith wanted to have sex with other men. I could see the interest developing as we worked together. I had sometimes commented on his interest, saying, "The idea of having sex with someone other than Alex seems less frightening and more appealing." Alex, locked into his own beliefs, did not consider that Keith might be changing and becoming more accepting of him. He thought that Keith was preparing to break up with him.

After proposing to open the relationship, Keith acknowledged that, as we had been examining and exploring sex and sexual values and the meaning of commitment, he had begun to have sexual fantasies about having sex with other men. Sure, he had fantasized about other men before, but this time it felt to him that the fantasies reflected his (realistic) wishes. Keith had been talking to friends who were polyamorous and had also listened to some podcasts he found on his own. Keith felt ready to explore CNM in the context of his ongoing relationship with Alex. Keith's interest in CNM made Alex anxious because he had never had to deal with a partner who was nonmonogamous. Alex was always the one creating space. We spent time discussing how his secrets had preserved some sense of power in the relationship. Now he had the same anxieties Keith had: "What if this doesn't work? What if someone else comes between us? What if Keith leaves me?"

We successfully avoided the pitfalls that would have come with letting Alex be the expert on polyamory. He had to acknowledge that he was not an expert, as he had never really practiced ethical or consensual nonmonogamy. So he and Keith needed to start from scratch to understand what would work for each of them as they opened their relationship. Once they reached this mutual decision, it was not actually that hard. Many of their friends in the gay community were polyamorous, and many of the couples they knew were not monogamous. They found a community of people they could talk with. This made their choice feel rather normal. Still, their friends' advice notwithstanding, it was important that Keith and Alex figure out together what might work for them as a couple.

After several months of having a lot of sex with a lot of different men, Keith and Alex settled into a slower and steadier pace that continued for at least the following year, during which time they continued in therapy. Alex had sex with other men when he went clubbing, which he did maybe once every month or two. Keith was not really into the club scene. He used apps to find someone to have sex with, mostly when he and Alex were apart from one another (work trips, family visits home, etc.). He liked the apps because he could spend some time flirting, allowing him to see if he was sexually interested before agreeing to meet.

Their sex life together resumed as an enjoyable part of their relationship. Did they talk about their other sexual experiences? Yes and no. They had a "don't ask, don't tell" policy, or more correctly framed, they had an "if you want to know, ask" policy. This did not mean they were obligated to supply sexual details if they preferred not to. Mostly, they did not ask or offer information about their other sexual experiences. They both seemed content to have sex with other men without emotional involvement or commitments. They agreed that if a relationship with someone else developed, they would talk with each other about it. During my time with them, this did not happen.

The decision to open a relationship is not a panacea. Alex continued to struggle with honesty, and with his impulse to be rebellious. Keith found that it was harder than he thought to let go of his desire to be a "good gay" and make his parents proud. He found that he missed important signals of problems or impending problems in his relationship with Alex, and when he did notice, he tended to rationalize the troubles away. Noticing what was going on (self and other) and communicating with each other was the focus of their last months of therapy.

"So, it's never going to be perfect," Keith said during our last session, "but if I know that and can see that and can talk about things that trouble me, we can make this work." He looked at Alex. "And I know," said Alex, "that if I need space or if I do or don't want to do something, I need to tell you. I know I don't have carte blanche to be a bad boy." Those words sounded something akin to marriage vows, or at least the small print of a marriage contract. But I am getting ahead of myself and clearly getting ahead of Keith and Alex, who have agreed that they will wait a while before considering marriage.

As they configured it, CNM was a positive experience for Keith and Alex. Their new relationship dynamic allowed Alex to enjoy being a "bad boy" at the clubs he went to, dancing and flirting and engaging in sex—most often group sex—if he wanted to. Interestingly, Keith mostly had sex with men he met on hookup apps when he and Alex were physically apart. He said that when Alex was around, he wanted to be with Alex. His occasional sex with others was very enjoyable and made him feel desirable. He also knew that it helped him maintain a sense of equilibrium; it did not feel right to him if Alex were the only one having sex with others.

KIM AND LAURA

Sex was very important to Kim. Growing up in Brooklyn with liberal parents, Kim's sexual orientation was celebrated and encouraged: "My parents were proud to be raising a lesbian." According to Kim, she had a lot of really great sex with a lot of really great women in her teens and 20s. There were no sexual experiences that she regretted, but there was no one person she wanted to settle down with either. Kim often had two or more girlfriends simultaneously, but she was open with all of them, and they each knew about her other relationships. Kim assumed that she would one day find the "right one" and settle down.

Laura was slow to discover her sexuality. She dated a lot of boys in high school and had a lot of heterosexual sex in college because it was the "thing to do." She regretted most, if not all, of those early sexual experiences because they brought her no particular pleasure and she often felt empty and used. In her mid-20s, Laura fell in love with Lydia and had satisfying sex for the first time in her life. The awareness of being gay brought Laura no particular angst, except that she was perplexed not to have known it before. In retrospect, she recognized her attraction to girls and women, but at the time, Laura just assumed she was not very sexual. Laura was devastated when Lydia broke up with her 18 months into the relationship. Laura became depressed, saw a psychiatrist, and went on antidepressant medication. She did not go to therapy.

Kim and Laura met through a dating app. Kim said she was attracted to Laura right away because she was quiet, smart, and kind. Laura said she was attracted to Kim because of her confidence and intelligence. The COVID-19 pandemic forced them into a decision: shelter together or go their separate ways. They sheltered together, driven by Kim's confidence that they could make this work as a monogamous couple.

Once they moved in together, their sex life deteriorated. While initially sex had been good (although not great, according to Kim), after moving in together, sex was disappointing at best. Laura wanted sex to happen quickly. She had to have sex in the dark. And she did not want Kim touching her. She was happy to stimulate Kim, and she was happy when Kim had an orgasm. Kim was not happy about any of it. As she later explained to me, "I really enjoy giving my partners pleasure, and I don't have that with Laura." In the isolation of the pandemic, Kim and Laura came to the decision to get married, thinking that the security of marriage would make sex better. After all, Laura often told Kim that she felt insecure in the relationship. She believed that the only reason they were together was that Kim did not want to be alone during the lockdown.

Kim and Laura came to see me 6 months after their wedding. As could be discerned from the camera angle, Kim felt that the focus of therapy should be on Laura and helping her be more comfortable with sex. Their attendance in therapy was sporadic; Laura and Kim would come for several sessions, and then they would say they needed to schedule a few weeks out because of work or other commitments. Laura appeared more willing to maintain weekly sessions. But when painful material came up in therapy, Kim would inevitably insist on a break. On the surface, it appeared that Kim was being protective of Laura, who was most often experiencing strong emotions in therapy. But I also thought that Kim was asking or insisting on a break from therapy because therapy was becoming too intimate for her.

I recommended individual therapy for both Laura and Kim, a recommendation they both accepted, but they also wanted to continue in couples therapy. Laura said, "I don't want to give up. This relationship is too important to me." Kim remained silent on that topic but agreed to continue the couples sessions.

Kim and Laura were not in a healthy relationship. On the urging of her individual therapist, Laura told Kim that the reason her relationship ended with Lydia was that the same pattern had developed in that relationship; Laura began to avoid sexual pleasure for herself, and Lydia lost interest. Laura apologized for not being truthful about her history and explained that she was now working on it. She and her therapist believed that it was the years of her having consensual but unwanted and unpleasant sex that had caused this effect. There was no abuse in her history, she assured Kim, and Laura expressed hope that sex with Kim would soon be good again.

Kim also shared insights from her individual therapy in our couples sessions. Kim said that she recognized she was being a caretaker for Laura and that she needed to stop doing this. She also said she had come to realize that she is polyamorous. Polyamory made sense to her; it appealed to her, it felt like her, and she had been happily polyamorous before she met Laura. Kim apologized to Laura, saying she had mistaken Laura's insecurity and dependence on her for love. She had mistakenly thought that monogamy was the ideal she should aspire to and that their emotional enmeshment was what monogamy must feel like. She was sorry she had been overly optimistic and unrealistic about herself in relationships. After tears and talking for several more sessions, Kim and Laura agreed to divorce.

Kim went on to practice solo polyamory, an approach to CNM that emphasizes autonomy and the freedom to choose relationships and often implies a commitment to living alone. Kim had two partners, with whom she had very intimate relationships, both sexually and emotionally. A third equally valued partner was primarily a sexual partner. Kim said that it felt healthier for her to spread her desire to please others over more than one relationship, and she also felt that her needs were met by her three partners in ways they could not or would not be by one. Kim was living alone with her two German shepherds ("See, I can't even be monogamous with a pet!"). This information came in a thank-you card Kim sent me. She told me that Laura had moved back home to the Midwest to be with her parents, and that is all Kim knew.

RESEARCH ON CONSENSUAL NONMONOGAMY

In *Polysecure*, Fern (2020) noted that the transition to CNM can bring up a lot of difficult feelings, including anxiety, insecurity, and jealousy. She notes that these feelings in and of themselves are not sufficient reasons to return to monogamy. The transition to CNM is not just having permission to have sex with other people; it is a fundamental shift in identity and in any preexisting relationship. Bumps are to be expected.

Taking a snapshot of the prevalence of polyamory finds estimates ranging between 0.6% and 5% of the adult population in North America. The low range of the estimate refers to endorsement of polyamory as an identity, whereas the higher estimate refers to polyamory defined as a relationship agreement. A much higher percentage, over 20%, of that same population of adult Americans, however, reports that they have practiced some form of polyamory across their lifetime (Rubel & Burleigh, 2020). Many people who practice CNM remain closeted, with 37% saying that they pass as monogamous when interacting with health care professionals. Of the 63% of their sample who did disclose their polyamory in a health care setting, Campbell et al. (2023) found that participants often felt misunderstood and judged. Commonly, health care practitioners were found to lack knowledge of polyamory, with many being curious and respectful, curious and disapproving, or curious and titillated. Polyamorous people report that they are subjected to unwanted and unnecessary medical procedures (e.g., testing for sexually transmitted infections [STIs] before being prescribed contraceptives) or they must listen to unwanted and unnecessary warnings: "You should reduce the number of partners you have." In other words, people who are polyamorous are often subjected to moralizing in the guise of medical advice. The ignorance about polyamory and the hypersexuality ascribed to polyamorous people is reinforced by the fact that most articles and studies on polyamory are published in sexology journals, as if family doctors, dentists, chiropractors, nurses, and general practice mental health professionals do not need to know about this *sexual* behavior (Campbell et al., 2023). The research is clear that, if anything, practicing CNM can reduce the risk of contracting or passing on an STI, as polyamorous people often get tested more often and tend to communicate more openly about STI status in comparison to their monogamous counterparts (Conley et al., 2015; Lehmiller, 2015).

In a review of the literature on relationship and sexual satisfaction, Gupta and her colleagues (2024) found that most studies reported that polyamorous people were as satisfied as or more satisfied than monogamous people in terms of their relationship happiness. Greater relationship satisfaction was found among older polyamorous adults (over 55), perhaps reflecting the benefit of shared connections and relationships with aging. In the few studies that reported lower relationship satisfaction among polyamorists, there was credible evidence that this was due to minority stress and internalized negativity about polyamory.

Gupta et al.'s (2024) comprehensive review also examined studies that compared different forms of polyamory, specifically hierarchical forms of polyamory versus nonhierarchical polyamory. In hierarchical forms of polyamory, there is a designated primary relationship, and other relationships are relegated to a secondary or tertiary status. In nonhierarchical forms of polyamory, there is no ranking, no veto powers, and no privileges (one notable example is called "relationship anarchy"). In nonhierarchical polyamory, no one can dictate what happens in another relationship, each relationship is left to develop on its own, and certain relationships must of necessity be prioritized at different times (e.g., a relationship in which you are raising children and sharing finances and property, or where a partner is ill). Across studies, relationship satisfaction is found to be higher in nonhierarchical relationships. Within hierarchical relationships, relationship satisfaction is found to be highest in the primary relationship, while more eroticism and higher sexual satisfaction are identified in the secondary relationships.

I did not have all this information when I began working with Anne and Scott, but what I did have was a willingness to learn about polyamory along with them.

ANNE AND SCOTT

Anne and Scott had been in couples therapy on and off for most of their marriage. It was helpful to them as they navigated Anne's depression and the impact it had on their parenting, family life, intimate relationship, and sex life. Anne's motivation to have sex varied depending on her depression, her level of guilt ("I am depriving Scott"), and her sense of obligation ("He does so much for me; I can at least have sex with him"). Anne had tried switching antidepressants and taking medications to improve her sex drive, and she and Scott experimented with sex toys, BDSM, and watching porn. None of it worked in the sense of sustaining a satisfying sexual connection. When they came to see me, they came with the express desire to talk about opening their relationship. More precisely, they wanted to talk about the possibility of Scott having sexual partners since Anne was not interested in having sex, although her depression was in remission. She felt emotionally healthy and grateful to have a career that she found fulfilling, a loving husband, a much-loved daughter (now living independently and far from her in Colorado), and a small but solid friendship group.

Anne was optimistic about opening up the marriage. She felt that she would finally be relieved of the burden of guilt she had carried for so long about not wanting to have sex with her husband. The sex that Anne envisioned Scott having might best be described as a *zipless fuck*, a term coined by Erica Jong (1973) in her novel *Fear of Flying*. A zipless fuck is sex without strings attached: no ulterior motives, no commitments, anonymous, and brief. Scott was a bit more circumspect. He felt that Anne had unrealistic expectations of what polyamory would be like. He knew he could not just have anonymous sex with strangers and never see them again; having an emotional connection with sex was key for him. He worried about how this would affect Anne's mental health and their marriage.

I was not an expert in polyamory, but Anne and Scott did not know whom to consult, and since I specialized in treating sexual problems, they thought I could help. We agreed that we would take this journey together. Anne and Scott felt confident that I was not going to promote a prepackaged version of polyamory but that I would work with them to find a relationship style that fit their needs.

Our first step was exploring their motivations for opening their marriage to see if they aligned. Anne was very clear that she wanted to be free of guilt, but as we discussed her feelings about Scott and how supportive he was and continued to be toward her, Anne said she truly wanted Scott to experience the happiness of an intimate sexual connection with someone. She just did not want to lose him. We would later learn that this feeling of pleasure in her partner's happiness with another person is called *compersion*. Anne wanted Scott to be happy. Her original idea of Scott having a series of zipless fucks was to soothe her anxiety, not to benefit Scott. Realizing this, Anne was able to realign her expectations.

Scott felt that he had a lot to give to relationships and was fully capable and excited by the prospect of giving to others. While Scott loved Anne, and while they shared so much history, a daughter, and a future (grandchildren, retirement, travel), he felt there were other life experiences (not just sexual experiences, but those too) that he longed for. Over the years, Scott had come to feel disillusioned with masculinity, and in his solo sexual experiences he began imagining himself, not as a woman, but not as a man either. He loved the idea of being, in his words, a "gender bender," and he wanted to play with gender expression sexually. "I just don't even get that" was Anne's response when Scott talked about wanting to be creative, playful, and exploratory in terms of sex and gender.

With the motivations clear, the next step was to find out more about polyamory. Scott took to the task and came to the next session with an abundance of knowledge. In retrospect, I should have been a bit more cautious, should have done more of my own research, and certainly should have noticed that Anne had not done any. The three of us were overly confident: Scott that he could handle multiple relationships, Anne that she would simply be happy for Scott, and I that my clinical judgment would be free of the privileged monogamy narrative in which I had been educated and trained (and which was reflected in the society in which we lived).

Rules

Anne accepted that Scott would be having intimate relationships and not just sex with other women (and perhaps with men). But she wanted to set a few ground rules: (a) The marriage needed to always come first because it was the primary relationship (if she felt that Scott was not prioritizing the marriage, she wanted him to know that she would call him on it); (b) Scott could have no dates within a 25-mile radius of their home and no partners who lived within 25 miles, or who might interact in any way with their friends and neighbors (Anne did not want to be embarrassed, she did not want people to think Scott was having an affair, and she did not want their daughter to be privy to this change in their relationship); and (c) She did not want to hear details, but she did want to know about Scott's relationships: who, when, and where. Implicit in this request was a veto power that Anne believed she should have over Scott's choices. Nevertheless, Scott thought these sounded like reasonable ground rules, so off he went to navigate the wonderful world of polyamory.

I am shaking my head incredulously at our collective naivete and my failure to recognize the cultural bias that led me to think that giving Scott's wife the power to dictate the parameters of his other relationships made sense. It took away Scott's right to manage his own relationships, and it certainly put his partners in the precarious position of having someone they have never met influence their lives. Anne's distance from Scott's other relationships made it highly likely that any veto powers she would exercise would be related to her own anxieties or to unresolved issues in her relationship with Scott. Managing anxiety and insecurity by trying to manage others is not a psychologically healthy strategy, whether we are talking about anxiety about sex, cleanliness, finances, or any number of issues.

All went exceedingly well in the beginning. Scott was meeting people in the polyamory community, and he felt welcomed and accepted. He went on many dates and finally settled into relationships with three women with whom he felt a connection. Going from one relationship to four in the space of a few months was overly ambitious, and Scott was unable to maintain his commitments to Anne. He failed to return phone calls to her (once when she had a flat tire), and in his excitement to go on a date, he neglected to sign some important forms their daughter needed to transfer bank funds, causing her to incur some heavy financial penalties. In violation of their agreement, he did have dates in a neighboring town, and mutual friends did run into him on one occasion. Scott also ran into trouble in his other relationships because he had not clearly communicated expectations.

So we returned to the drawing board, with Scott having one other relationship (with Margaret) in addition to his relationship with Anne. "I think this is more manageable for me" was Scott's assessment. I have come to learn that the term *polysaturated* stands for the point at which the polyamorous person has all the relationships they can handle and has neither the time nor the emotional energy for more (Sheff, 2021). At this point in his life as a polyamorist, Scott's number was two (Anne and Margaret). It would later increase to three, but we are getting ahead of ourselves.

Hierarchies

The important issue that was overlooked in Scott and Anne's journey was that they were relying on rules to make sure that Scott balanced his commitments. The rules made Anne feel that she had some power in what was happening, and yet those rules did not help. Emotions are not easily governed by restrictions. Scott felt terrible for letting Anne down, and for not being there for their daughter. But more than being polysaturated, Scott and Anne had not truly considered what they needed from each other emotionally, nor had they fully grasped how hard this would be. Apart from discussing their transition to CNM with me, neither Scott nor Anne had anyone to confide in about their struggles.

Instead of relying on rules, Anne and Scott began to explore what level of commitment was needed in their relationship and how that commitment could be expressed. We did not know it at the time, but Anne and Scott were moving from a prescriptive hierarchy to a descriptive one. Initially they were trying to prescribe how their relationship and Scott's other relationships would coexist. They were prescribing the primacy of their marriage and relegating the other relationships to secondary or tertiary status. No wonder some of Scott's partners balked at how he was attempting to manage them. When hierarchies are prescriptive, the partner in the primary relationship may have veto power over the course of another relationship, including ending it. Descriptive hierarchies make room for different types of commitments. What evolved for Scott was the commitment he had to Anne, which was to share parenting, finances, certain familial and social obligations, and a high level of emotional intimacy and honesty.

Another of Scott's relationships became important because it was in this relationship that he felt free to explore the breadth of his gender expression. He was able to explore his body in different manifestations, to explore sexuality in ways that masculinity did not allow. Scott also had a third relationship. This relationship was important to him because he felt part of a larger community of artists and intellectuals with this woman as his partner.

Scott's marriage to Anne was his most important relationship; it was primary. Instead of Anne being able to dictate how Scott's other relationships would work (e.g., "I'm not comfortable with you sleeping over for two nights; I think one is enough. I don't think it's appropriate for you to meet her children; I think it sends the wrong message."), Scott learned to manage his relationships by accepting responsibility for prioritizing his relationship with Anne (rather than having her dictate his priorities). Rather than trying valiantly to please three women, Scott learned to balance his own priorities ("I'm not comfortable meeting your children quite yet; let's hold off on that. I have been away from Anne for several weekends; I'm going to say no to sleeping over."). Scott and Anne learned to check in with each other and discuss how to best manage their relationship so that their needs were met. As much as Anne may have thought she would not have to do much work in her relationship, she found, to the contrary, that she and Scott had to communicate more, not less, about their relationship needs, expectations, and boundaries.

Jealousy

Anne frequently struggled, especially in the early days of their open marriage, with feelings of being left out and jealous. She worried that Scott would love one of his new partners more than he loved her; she compared herself to his other partners and found herself wanting ("I'm a loser; I just sit at home and do nothing"). The urge that Anne had was to ask Scott to curtail his activities so that she would not have these feelings ("Maybe you can wait until I'm more ready"). However, these feelings seemed to be those one would expect in this situation. I encouraged Anne to sit with the feelings and to regulate her emotional state in ways other than by asking Scott to do things or sacrifice for her. This was a pattern that had been established during her depression of course, but it is not unusual in monogamous relationships where one partner feels the need to be everything for the other.

Anne used time in therapy to talk about her feelings of inadequacy and jealousy. Scott listened and empathized, but (with a lot of help at first) he refrained from trying to fix things for her. Anne has not had a relapse of her depression. Her mood continues to be stable. Anne has recognized that she is happiest at home, and that does not make her a "loser." She is getting more engaged in hobbies she felt she did not have time for before, namely, gardening and knitting. She is an avid reader and has joined a book club, so not all of her activities are solo. Anne derives a lot of pleasure and self-worth from her career and no longer feels guilty for taking time from Scott to work. She and Scott enjoy going to basketball games and other sports events together, activities that they enjoyed earlier in their relationship.

Anne and Scott are still in therapy, although they now come about once a month. They find it helpful to process the continuing challenges they face and the mix of emotions that they could never have predicted before. Both Anne and Scott agree that the polyamory they practice has strengthened their relationship. They feel more connected to each other and more satisfied with their lives in general.

THE PURPLE-HAIRED UNICORN

Back in Chapter 2, I introduced you to Ellen, a polyamorous woman who was fearful of a recurrence of depression due to the loneliness of losing connection with important partners after she relocated with her husband from New York to New Jersey. You do not need to flip the pages back to Chapter 2; I have just told you what is necessary for you to know about her now. In a weird twist of fate, and further proof that truth is often stranger than fiction, I recently ran into Ellen while we were both hiking in a state park, and she caught me up on her life. I remembered Ellen well. She struggled to be her authentic self in many of her relationships—with her husband, her colleagues at work, and her family. She attributed her sense of disconnection to having to hide significant aspects of herself in order to be liked and accepted. In therapy, she talked about not knowing herself well and was constantly questioning herself. At the point where the story left off in Chapter 2, Ellen was wondering whether she wanted to renegotiate some of the boundaries with her husband and what to make of her awareness of her attraction to women. When Ellen left therapy, she was no longer worried about her depression returning and was feeling less lonely, having made friends and beginning a relationship with an emotionally available and sexually attractive man.

Fast-forward almost 3 years and relocate us to a wooded trail where three people stop to admire and pet my dog, Mika, an engaging and spirited Coton de Tuléar. "Dr. Hall? Dr. Hall!" I looked at the woman with the bright purple hair and recognized Ellen. "I thought it was you! Dr. Hall, this is my boyfriend, Matt, and my girlfriend, Hannah, Matt's wife." After we said our hellos, Ellen asked if she could walk with me a bit to catch me up on her life. I happily agreed, and Matt and Hannah went ahead. Here is some of what Ellen told me:

> When I left therapy, I was in a pretty good place, and even when Vic [the man she was seeing] broke up with me, I was still okay. But in my head, I kept thinking about being authentic, to myself mostly—you know, what we worked on pretty much every session. After the breakup, I stopped looking for a boyfriend and stayed home more, which annoyed my husband. He said I was interfering in his relationships—and I was! But not because I wanted to ruin them; I wanted to be in them. I liked the women he was involved with, and I wanted to be involved with them too—sexually and intimately. For once, I didn't just accept what someone told me about me. I wasn't trying to break his relationships up, as he thought; I was trying to be in them. Turns out that my husband didn't want that. But other people do want me! I've been with Matt and Hannah for over a year now. I'm so happy.

Ellen also said that she introduced Matt and Hannah to me as husband, wife, boyfriend, and girlfriend partly to shock me but also to tell me quickly that there was more to the story.

> We are all equals in this relationship. We usually just say we are partners and let others figure it out. It may be time for lawyers soon. I want to get divorced so the three of us can buy a house. And then the paperwork about medical power of attorney and all that will have to happen. Too bad we can't all three be married.

I told Ellen I was writing a book and that her story (well disguised) was in an early chapter. Ellen was pleased: "I made it in your book!" So I asked her if I could ask her some more detailed questions—questions I likely would not have asked had I not been in the middle of writing. Ellen was enthusiastic, and she joked, "You know this goes right to the heart of my wanting to feel important, right?" Ellen met Matt and Hannah at a party thrown by a polyamorous friend. Ellen liked them right away. They were a married couple but were interested in adding a third.

At this point, some definitions are in order. A *throuple* or a *triad* is a form of polyamory comprised of three people. If it is a closed system, then it functions very similarly to monogamy, in that the members do not date or have sex with anyone outside of the triad. However, triads need not be closed to others; they can be open.

A triad is just one type of *polycule*. *Polycule* is a more general term for a network of people who are intimate and sexual with one or more other individuals in the group. If these definitions sound vague and incomplete to you, they are. People who are polyamorous negotiate (and renegotiate) relationship boundaries that work for them. So, when inquiring about polyamorous relationships, you will have to ask, "What does that look like for you?" Fern (2020) writes that "there is no one right way to practice CNM and it is more of a 'create your own relationship' than a one-size-fits-all approach" (p. 109).

Being in a triad or a throuple was not something that Ellen had previously considered, but the more time she spent with Matt and Hannah, the more this felt to her like an authentic way of being in a relationship. It felt right.

> It's the first time for all of us, being in a throuple, so we have to decide on the boundaries that work for us. We talk a lot. We're actually surprisingly monogamous, if that makes sense; we've decided that we don't need the drama of other sex partners, and a larger polycule feels like way too much work.

Ellen went on to tell me that they have agreed on no outside sex partners; it is just the three of them, and sex occurs in different configurations: Sometimes the three of them and sometimes two will pair off.

> My feelings of being left out and feeling unimportant get triggered a lot, but I know what they are, where they come from, and that they will pass. It's getting easier, but it's still not completely easy. Every Sunday we have Muffin Morning Meeting, kind of a state-of-the-union check-in. I might find that hard [she joked], but I really love the muffins we take turns baking.

Ellen was still teaching math, and once she started looking more like herself, she realized that having a purple-haired female math teacher was something the prestigious private school was actually quite proud of. "I'm in almost all the marketing brochures," she told me. Ellen also explained that she was a *unicorn*, a term for the rare bisexual woman who is interested in being in a relationship with a man and a bisexual woman.

I have greatly condensed our conversation for the purposes of this book, but I was very happy to have encountered Ellen, to see that she was happy, and to see that she was continuing her therapy on her own: "Dr. Hall, you are often in my head. I often ask myself, 'What would Dr. Hall say?' The answer usually is to trust myself."

SUMMARY

Consensual nonmonogamy is an umbrella term for relationship constellations that differ from monogamous couplings. *Swinging*, *open marriage*, and *polyamory* are some of the terms that fall under this umbrella. More precisely defining these different constellations is difficult, as they are uniquely tailored to what works now for the people involved. Boundaries around emotional and sexual intimacy are negotiated and renegotiated in CNM relationships.

The role of the therapist is similar to that in other therapeutic endeavors: to help our patients better understand themselves so that they can make choices that are right for them. Helping our patients understand their sexuality is crucial when the choices they face involve intimate and sexual relationships. Opening an existing relationship to others requires thoughtful communication between existing partners as well as new partners.

As the cases in this chapter illustrate, there are different motivations for exploring CNM, and different outcomes may result from that exploration. CNM is not associated with psychopathology and, in fact, can result in very high levels of relationship satisfaction. Monogamy does not have a monopoly on intimacy. The rising interest in CNM makes it likely that we will encounter patients who are in nontraditional relationships or who want our help as they navigate the transition to CNM.

CONCLUSION

Sex Is Not a Specialty

Talking about sex in psychotherapy should not be a specialty. It should be a core competency, like listening, empathy, and having ethical boundaries. Every therapist needs to have the ability to talk about sex in psychotherapy. As a therapist, acquiring this skill requires that you have an understanding of the fundamental models of human sexuality and an awareness and acceptance of the diversity of sexual expressions and experiences that our patients will bring to therapy. You do not need to be an expert on all things sexual, and in truth, you do not even have to be very sexual yourself. There have been times in my career when I was just not very interested in sex: I had just suffered a breakup, I was stressed and busy, or I had just had a baby, and then another one! And yet, I was still an effective therapist, talking about sex with my patients. I was still interested in their sexual concerns because it was their sexuality that I was talking about, not mine. Talking about sex in psychotherapy means that you understand that sex is fundamental to a sense of identity and to how our patients relate to themselves and to others. It is also quite often implicated in the problems that our patients experience.

Frankly, we need to talk about sex in psychotherapy because our patients want to talk about sex. They want to understand why they make the choices they do and why they are experiencing the problems that confound them.

https://doi.org/10.1037/0000483-012
Talking About Sex in Psychotherapy: A Guide for Every Therapist, by K. S. K. Hall

And we need to talk about sex in psychotherapy because not talking about it allows our patients to hide important parts of themselves. We need to give our patients opportunities to be honest about what they most commonly lie about in therapy: sex. We need to talk about sex in psychotherapy to help patients unburden themselves from the shame they may carry. We need to talk about sex in psychotherapy because doing so provides another perspective on the psychology of our patients. Sex mirrors and magnifies important intrapersonal and interpersonal dynamics. The cases in this book illustrate how talking about sex in psychotherapy helps move therapy forward.

I have always had a general practice alongside my sex therapy practice. But I know that many of my general practice patients choose to see me because of my background in sex therapy. People come to sex therapists for various sex-adjacent problems because they believe they will not be judged, they will be understood, and sex will be discussed. Many of these sex and sex-related problems are described in this book: infidelity, pornography use, loneliness, difficulty finding or keeping a partner, and processing shameful or traumatic experiences. People who belong to a sexual minority group (because of the sex they like [e.g., kinky sex], their choice of partner[s] [same or opposite gender, nonbinary], or their identity [gay, bisexual, polyamorous]) often choose to see sex therapists, even when the presenting problem is not sexual. Being identified as a sex therapist is interpreted by the help-seeking public, especially by sexual minorities, as meaning a nonjudgmental professional who understands sexual diversity and who can talk about sex without pathologizing people's sexual choices. Of course, I hope that one day the help-seeking public will know that every psychotherapist is (or should be!) nonjudgmental, understanding, and capable of talking about sex without pathologizing. When this day comes, it will not mean that sex therapy has outlived its usefulness. Far from it.

The more people talk about sex and sexual problems, the more likely it is that therapists will be needed to help patients navigate their difficulties. The question of what separates sex therapy from other therapies is, therefore, an important and valid question, especially if you are considering becoming a sex therapist.

THE SEPARATE TREATMENT OF SEXUAL PROBLEMS

How did we come to a separate therapy for sexual problems? After all, Sigmund Freud, who famously pioneered the talking cure, did not think that sexual problems required a different or unique treatment approach. Freud

(1905) attributed sexual problems, as he did all types of mental illness, to unresolved psychic conflicts that could be resolved with insight-oriented analysis. Following in the footsteps of psychoanalysis, many subsequent schools of therapy, particularly psychodynamically oriented approaches, continued to adhere to the belief that sexual problems were caused by underlying psychopathology and that once the psychological, relational, or emotional issues were addressed, sex would naturally improve. Cognitive behavior therapists, on the other hand, were already practicing a symptom-focused approach to treatment when Masters and Johnson's (1966, 1970) research made a strong case for attending to sexual problems in their own right. While there is no data on this, it is very plausible that those cognitive behavior therapists who were already comfortable talking about sex were drawn to the new field of sex therapy.

Newly minted sex therapists were getting comfortable talking about erections, vaginal lubrication, pain occurring during penile–vaginal penetration, the timing of ejaculation, and toe-tingling orgasms or lack thereof—sexual problems that could be resolved with targeted behavioral interventions. For sex therapists, sex is not a symptom of a deeper conflict; rather, sex is the problem. Problematic sex could and should be directly addressed and replaced with pleasurable sex via a series of exercises designed to alleviate performance anxiety.

THE EXPANSION OF SEX THERAPY

These siloed approaches to the treatment of sexual problems continued for decades. Sex therapists formed their own societies and associations, published journals, and held workshops specifically devoted to sex research and the practice of sex therapy. The emergence of sexual medicine in the 1990s required sex therapy to reckon with the biological mechanisms that were now frequently implicated in sexual dysfunctions. Pills and injections helped men achieve and maintain erections; medications helped delay ejaculation; and creams, surgeries, pelvic floor exercises, and vaginal dilators helped alleviate painful sex. Sometimes sexual medicine was needed to help the body function, while sex therapy was needed to help the individual or couple experience their functionality as pleasure. The treatment of sexual problems was becoming an interdisciplinary affair, with sex therapists attending to the psychological and relational concerns and medical professionals evaluating and treating medical or biological issues (Meana & Hall, 2024).

In the decades following Masters and Johnson, sex therapists began to notice something important. They observed that the patients seeking sex therapy were not presenting with performance anxiety, or at least not solely presenting with performance anxiety. Instead, sex therapists were seeing patients with histories of trauma, complicated medical and psychological profiles, cancer that interfered with sexual functioning, depression and anxiety and their medications that diminished sexual desire and function, and sexually transmitted infections that required shame-inducing negotiations in intimate relationships. Sex therapists also saw patients whose sexuality was affected by their neurodiversity, physical and intellectual disability, and aging, illness, and addictions. Consequently, behaviorally focused exercises were insufficient to meet the needs of this patient population.

In reality, Masters and Johnson's approach to sex therapy was relatively short lived as a comprehensive treatment approach. Helen Singer Kaplan (1974), who amended the human sexual response cycle to include the desire phase, also noted that sometimes the treatment of sexual problems required a deeper exploration of guilt, trauma, attachment disorders, and problematic relationship dynamics. Following Kaplan's lead, sex therapists (who are, after all, first trained in some other discipline: psychology, clinical social work, or counseling) brought their therapeutic orientations to the practice of sex therapy. These included existential, Gestalt, humanistic, object relations, systemic, emotion-focused, and third-wave cognitive behavior therapies like mindfulness. Essentially, Kaplan offered an open invitation to therapists of all theoretical orientations to apply their knowledge to what might be causing or maintaining sexual problems. However, not many therapists opted in, so sex therapy maintained its identity as a specialized treatment approach, despite looking not a whole lot like the specialty treatment that Masters and Johnson envisioned (Meana & Hall, 2024).

SEX THERAPY AS A DISTINCT PRACTICE

What distinguishes sex therapists from other therapists is threefold: Sex therapists recognize the importance of sex in the lives and relationships of people, have a high level of comfort with sexuality and are therefore comfortable discussing sexual issues in psychotherapy, and have the ability, when doing therapy, to simultaneously attend to underlying issues and the problematic sex that brought the individual or couple to therapy in the first place. Recognition of the importance of sex and comfort with sexuality will lead therapists to get training in human sexuality, which will increase comfort levels as well as therapists' ability to directly address sexual problems in treatment. Therapists who are uncomfortable with sex may self-select out of training and sexuality courses. Thus, the gap widens.

Many people assume that what is unique about sex therapy is that it comprises highly effective, time-limited, specialized interventions. It is true that sex therapy often involves the application of targeted treatments that are largely based on learning principles. Systematic desensitization, a standard behavioral intervention, is a core component of sex therapy. Many sex therapy homework assignments involve refraining from anxiety-producing sexual activities and then working through a graded hierarchy of sexual interactions with a focus on pleasure rather than anxiety. Sensate focus is one application of desensitization, as is the use of dilators for women with pain or fear of pain with penetrative sex.

Sex therapy is not just a compilation of sexual exercises prepackaged for specific dysfunctions. This mistaken belief has led to poor-quality outcomes in therapy. In some circumstances, the misapplication of sex therapy techniques is a way for therapists to minimize their own discomfort while attempting to help individuals or couples with sexual problems.

A CAUTIONARY TALE ABOUT SEX EXERCISES

Ginny and Collin came to see me in crisis. Ginny had recently discovered a long-term affair (4 years) that Collin had been having with a coworker. The discovery of the affair coincided with Ginny receiving a diagnosis of multiple sclerosis (MS). "Just when I need him the most, I find out that I can't trust him." Ginny was devastated. Collin was full of guilt, remorse, and self-recrimination: "It was only sexual. You're the love of my life." Ginny needed to know why Collin had an affair; she wanted to trust him again but could not understand his betrayal. Apparently, it all started with a badly handled treatment for premature ejaculation. Here is the story as I came to understand it:

Ginny and Collin had seen a couples therapist early in their marriage. Their sex life was disappointing, and they wanted help with Collin's premature ejaculation (PE). Collin ejaculated within about 30 seconds of having intercourse with Ginny. The therapist gave them a sheet of paper with instructions for stop/start, a sex therapy technique used to treat PE that involves stopping sexual stimulation prior to ejaculation and letting arousal subside before starting again. This sequence is repeated as needed to help men focus on their sexual arousal and prolong the length of time they can sustain moderate levels of sexual excitement without ejaculating. Ginny and Collin tried the stop/start exercises but had no success. Collin continued to ejaculate within seconds of having intercourse.

The therapist then suggested they try the squeeze technique, which was a variation of stop/start; instead of just stopping stimulation, either Collin or Ginny should squeeze Collin's penis where the shaft joins the head and continue the pressure until the urge to ejaculate passes. Ginny and Collin tried the squeeze technique just once. They found the whole process awkward and uncomfortable, so they stopped going to therapy and continued to have the disappointing sex they had before: rushing through foreplay to get to intercourse in the hopes that Collin could last at least a few seconds before he ejaculated. Ginny concluded that she just had to put up with having mediocre sex, and she tried to make the best of it to avoid making Collin feel bad.

Over the following years, however, Ginny lost all desire for sex with Collin. She continued to masturbate and enjoy sex on her own, but only very infrequently did she have sex with Collin. Collin was hurt by Ginny's lack of interest and had no idea it was because of his PE. He had tried the sex therapy exercises, and they did not work. What more could he do? Ginny had assured him many times that it was all right and did not matter to her. So why the loss of desire? Collin surmised that Ginny must just not be that interested in sex. But Collin was lonely and missed having sex.

Collin did not experience PE with his affair partner for the simple reason that they did not have intercourse. Instead of rushing through foreplay, they touched, caressed, and brought each other to orgasm with their hands and mouth. Collin enjoyed the sex he was having with his affair partner. It never occurred to him to have sex with Ginny in the same way because he thought Ginny was not interested. Now, Ginny felt cheated out of having a good sex life. She would have loved to have had the kind of sex Collin had with his affair partner. With the prospect looming of physical decline due to her MS, including the loss of orgasm, her grief was immense.

It was not only PE that caused the affair or the loneliness in their marriage or Ginny's sadness. But Collin's PE was instrumental in setting in motion a series of events that Ginny and Collin did not know how to navigate. The fact that they thought they had tried and failed at a treatment for PE precluded them from seeking help elsewhere. The therapist was likely well meaning in her attempt to help the couple with their sexual problems. She knew enough to understand that there were behavioral interventions for PE, but she did not know enough to know that was not enough.

TALKING ABOUT SEX WITH PSYCHOTHERAPISTS: A PLEA FOR INTEGRATION

Graduate school is where we grow and develop as therapists. We seek out professors who mentor us and internships where we learn the skills necessary to begin to practice. But there is very scant education regarding human sexuality and even less training on how to treat sexual problems in our graduate school curricula. Most therapists who eventually become sex therapists get their sexuality education and sex therapy training in postgraduate courses and continuing education workshops and seminars (Meana & Hall, 2024; Zeglin et al., 2024). This means that only those therapists with a (preexisting) interest and comfort in human sexuality will opt for further training in sexuality. Therefore, we are missing an opportunity to help aspiring therapists become more comfortable with the topic of sexuality such that they, too, might seek out additional training in sex therapy. If we are to integrate an understanding of the importance of attending to sexual issues in psychotherapy, we need to start early in the training trajectory of therapists.

In addition to talking about sex in psychotherapy training programs and graduate schools, we have to talk about sex with other psychotherapists. We need to publish in each other's journals, attend and present at each other's conferences, and ask for consultation and supervision from each other. And what we talk about when we talk about sex is also important. Almost half of the sexuality-related articles published in counseling journals are focused on sexual identity, leaving notable gaps regarding sexual pleasure, sexual functioning, and sexual lifestyles (Zeglin et al., 2019). The American Association of Sex Educators, Counselors and Therapists (AASECT, n.d.) outlines areas of core competencies for sex therapists, which include anatomy/physiology, sexual functioning, sociocultural and familial factors, developmental sexuality, intimacy skills, diversity, and ethics. These could serve as a template for graduate school curricula as well as for journals and professional conferences seeking to expand the scope of their offerings.

As more therapists become comfortable talking about sex with their patients, there will still be a need for specialized practices. Some patients and their situations are highly complex and require the experience and expertise of a seasoned sex therapist. Other patients have sexual problems that require a level of knowledge not every therapist possesses. There are sex therapists who specialize in the impact of cancer and cancer treatments on patients' sexuality, while others work in the context of fertility treatment programs or sexual pain clinics. Additionally, some sex therapists focus on special populations: young people, sexual minority groups, elder people, people with disabilities, members of religious groups, and so on.

AN ETHICAL IMPERATIVE

Talking about sex in psychotherapy is, importantly, an ethical matter. There is credible evidence that talking about sex in psychotherapy will improve patient honesty, thereby improving the effectiveness of the therapy. There is credible evidence that talking about sex will also help alleviate a major source of our patients' shame, which will therefore also improve the efficacy and outcomes of the therapy process (Farber et al., 2019). How can we then ethically not talk about sex in psychotherapy?

Talking about sex in psychotherapy is also a matter of access and inclusion. If sexuality is a specialty, then getting access to treatment for sexual concerns and problems will be difficult, perhaps especially for marginalized groups. Given that therapists have the skills to incorporate the treatment of many sexual issues into their general psychotherapy practice, is it not ethical for them to do so if it expands access to care?

People come to therapy to understand themselves more fully and to resolve whatever issues they are struggling with. Sometimes—often, almost always—they need and want to talk about their sexuality. Every therapist should have the clinical skills to talk about sex in psychotherapy, to integrate information about patients' sexuality into a comprehensive and deeper understanding of the person seeking help, and to intervene helpfully when patients struggle with sexual issues. It is my hope that this book has provided the inspiration and the blueprint for these ongoing endeavors.

Appendix A

WOMEN'S SEXUAL AROUSAL

In my lifetime, women have been, if not ashamed, then certainly not proud of their genitals. I grew up in an era when we were being sold feminine deodorant sprays. Today, cosmetic surgeries are marketed to women to improve the appearance of their vulvas. These surgeries are designed to make labia more symmetrical and vaginas tighter. And although I wonder just who is looking and judging the symmetry of women's labia, I know that it is often women's own anxieties that fuel the industries, which then further fuel our anxieties. In the spirit of trying to contribute to healthier and more positive attitudes, I offer the following empirically based and sex-positive description of women's sexual anatomy and response. Unless otherwise referenced, the anatomical and physiological information comes from Levay and Valente's (2006) textbook on human sexuality.

TERMINOLOGY

First, let us get some terms down. Women's genitals are often referred to simply as their "vaginas." This reductionist term relegates the complexity of women's sexual anatomy to the one structure that serves (sexually) to accommodate a penis and (reproductively) to deliver a baby. The correct term for female external genitalia is *vulva*. The vulva includes the mons veneris (mountain of Venus), sometimes known as mons pubis, or pubic mound. It is made of fatty tissue and serves to cushion the pubic area during sex. It may not be considered the sexiest part of a woman's body, but it is important—otherwise, ouch. Other parts of the vulva include the labia majora (outer lips) and labia minora (inner lips) and the clitoris and the clitoral hood as well as the vaginal opening. I will say more about each soon.

AROUSAL

A woman must be ready and willing to engage in sex, with herself or with someone (or some others) of her choosing in order for these physical responses to occur and to be accompanied by the subjective experience of pleasure.

In a nonaroused state, the walls of the vagina are relaxed and touching, and the inner labia are folded together, shielding the opening of the vagina from the outside world. Think of drapes being drawn to keep out the early morning sunlight. The inner lips are usually referred to as the labia minora, and as the Pulitzer Prize–winning journalist and author Natalie Angier (2000) describes them, are "the exquisite inner origami of flesh that enfolds the vagina and nearby urethral opening" (p. 54).

When a woman is stimulated (by fantasies or by touch), blood flows to the genitals. Many women will experience this as a subtle but perceptible feeling of warmth and perhaps some tingling of the genitals as the blood reaches them. Some women will identify this feeling as desire: the mental wish for sexual stimulation combined with subtle suggestive sensations. Other women will think that this is arousal. Neither is wrong. Many women do not distinguish sexual desire from the early stages of sexual arousal (Graham et al., 2004). So while some women think of sexual desire as a motivational state or an intention, others will not recognize sexual desire unless it is accompanied by some physical manifestation of arousal.

As stimulation continues, blood flows to the genital area and the vagina begins to lubricate. Vaginal lubrication is a very early sign of arousal and not an indication that a woman is ready (physically or mentally) for intercourse. If there is penetrative sex at this point, it is likely not to be painful (it may be uncomfortable), but it is not likely to be sexually satisfying. It takes a little longer for the accumulation of blood in the vulva to reach a point where the labia (both inner and outer lips), the clitoris, and the pelvic floor become engorged and, therefore, cushiony. The vaginal canal expands, and the uterus tips forward and up, which allows space for a penis. This is called vaginal tenting or ballooning. At this point women will often feel a desire for penetrative sex (fingers, penis, dildo).

The elasticity of the vagina is, of course, well-known to all who understand how most babies are delivered into this world. Angier (2000) is also a fan:

> But the vagina, now there's a Rorschach with legs. You can make of it practically anything you want, need or dread. . . . It is a four- to five-inch-long tunnel that extends at a forty-five-degree angle from the labia to the doughnut-shaped cervix. It is a pause between the declarative sentence of the outside world and the mutterings of the viscera. . . . It is the most obliging of passageways,

> one that will stretch to accommodate travelers of any conceivable dimension, whether they are coming (penises, speculums) or going (infants). (p. 51)

The outer third of the vagina is innervated and sensitive to touch. The deeper two thirds of the vaginal canal are sensitive to pressure. During arousal, the outer third of the vagina narrows to fit snugly around a penis (or dildo or fingers), creating a pleasurable sensation for the woman and her partner (but not the dildo, which has no feelings). Breast tissue may also become warm and engorged by increased blood flow. Nipples may or may not become erect. And then, perhaps most significantly for women's pleasure, the clitoris becomes engorged and erect as well. I will defer again to Angier (2000) to poetically describe this process:

> The clitoral glans is the wick of Eros, the site where the 8000 nerve fibers are threshed together into a proper little brain. . . . The shaft has relatively few nerves, but it is threaded through with thousands of blood vessels, allowing it to swell during arousal and push the head ever higher. Further facilitating the great clitoral expansion are two bundles of erectile tissue wrapped in a muscle called the bulbs of the vestibule, which help impel blood headward. Thus insanguinated, the passionate clitoris inflates to twice the size of the clitoris supine. (pp. 65–66)

The clitoris is more than the glans, or head, that "sits proudly, may be a bit smugly, beneath its A-lined roof, a hood formed by the junction of the inner labia" (Angier, 2000, p. 64). As Figure A.1 shows, the clitoris also has a shaft and legs, or *crura* (*crus* in the singular), as they are referred to in the scientific literature, that extend two to three and a half inches down and toward the vaginal opening, following the lines of the labia minora (Cass, 2004). It is believed that while most women need some stimulation of the glans for orgasm, for some women, the crura of the clitoris may extend far enough so that the friction of intercourse will provide stimulation to the clitoris (the crura) and thus an orgasm may happen.

ORGASM

An orgasm is quite simply a reflex reaction that occurs when, at some point of sexual excitement, the body reverses direction. Blood flow (which has engorged the vulva and created warmth, a feeling of fullness, and perhaps some throbbing due to raised blood pressure) and the muscular tension that has been building (which may have extended beyond the vulva so that fingers and toes might also feel taut) reach a peak. This reversal of these processes that have been building feels like a release, and this is an orgasm.

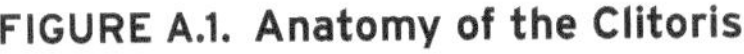
FIGURE A.1. Anatomy of the Clitoris

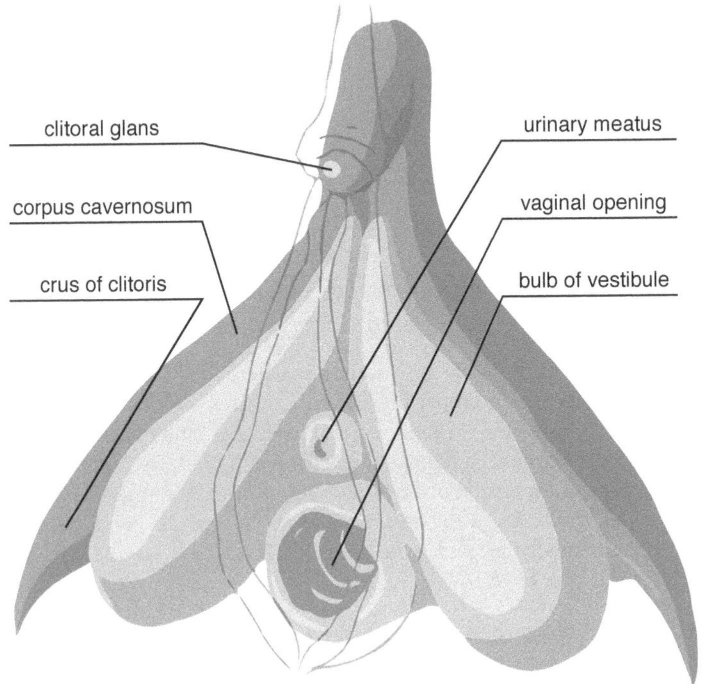

Note. From *Internal Anatomy of the Human Vulva, Focusing on the Anatomy and Location of the Clitoris* [Figure], by Amphis, Marnanel, & Xeror, 2017, Wikimedia Commons (https://commons.wikimedia.org/wiki/File:Clitoris_Anatomy.svg). CC BY-SA 4.0.

It cannot be willed or forced into happening. It is the natural response to the buildup of arousal. If an orgasm does not occur, it is likely due to insufficient stimulation, the interference of anxiety, distraction, or other mental/emotional states that inhibit arousal.

FEMALE EJACULATION AND THE G-SPOT

The G-spot, or Grafenberg spot, is a matter of some scientific contention, with researchers and clinicians debating its existence and questioning the occurrence of female ejaculation. For clinicians and for our female patients, the important point is that women should not spend inordinate amounts of time or energy searching for a G-spot, nor should they have to defend their belief that they, in fact, have such a spot of pleasurable sensitivity on the anterior wall of their vagina. Women who have never expelled fluid through their urethra during orgasm need not try to do so, nor worry that they might. Women who feel proud of ejaculating may continue to take pride. Some women worry that they might lose control and release urine during orgasm. This is a different story, and an anxiety that can be resolved by encouraging women to find the time to empty their bladder before sex.

OUCH!

Sex should not hurt. Ever. Pain means something is wrong. Women should pay attention to their pain and have their pain attended to. Pain may indicate that some or all of the wonderful ways their body protects them from painful intercourse (the vasocongestion that provides cushioning, the vaginal lubrication that prevents vaginal tearing, the tenting or ballooning to make room for the penis) are not happening, because there has not been enough, or good enough, sexual stimulation.

Pain that occurs deep in the vagina may be due to the penis hitting the cervix when there is deep penetration and thrusting. The solution is to switch positions so that the penis cannot reach the cervix. Rear entry, or what is colloquially called "doggie style," is one option.

Many women from traditional cultures or backgrounds who were admonished to guard their virginity, or who were told or taught that intercourse hurts, may become fearful of pain with intercourse. They tense their muscles in dread anticipation, and then, in a self-fulfilling prophecy, the pain occurs. Vaginal penetration with muscles clenched, especially the muscles of the pelvic floor, hurts.

Some women have spastic muscles in their pelvic floor from back injuries or other medical issues and may require pelvic floor physical therapy to address and relax the muscles so that intercourse will not hurt.

Pain may indicate the presence of an infection or a dermatological condition. It may also be due to a condition called *vulvodynia*, which refers to chronic or episodic pain in the vulva. When the pain is localized at the opening to the vagina, the condition is called *vestibulodynia* (referring to the pain at the entrance or vestibule). If the pain occurs only when there is touch or pressure applied to the area, the condition is referred to as *provoked vestibulodynia*. The pain is often described as burning or stinging, and it will, of course, interfere with sexual activities and sexual pleasure. There is no known cause for vulvodynia, but some combination of the following issues may be implicated: nerve damage or injury, previous infections, surgeries, hormonal fluctuations, and genetic predisposition.

MENOPAUSE

Levels of estrogen decrease around menopause (defined as the cessation of menstruation for one full year). This drop in estrogen can lead to vaginal dryness and thinning of the vaginal walls. There is less lubrication and decreased elasticity of the vaginal walls. The vagina may also shorten and become tighter, especially at the entrance. These changes can lead to pain (and sometimes tearing and bleeding of vaginal tissue) during sexual intercourse (North American Menopause Society, n.d.b). In such cases, a gynecologist may recommend some combination of the following: hormone therapy, pelvic floor physical therapy, vaginal moisturizers, lubricants, or regular exercises with vaginal dilators.

Another concern during menopause, however, is the decrease in desire that many women may experience. Hormone therapy may address this decrease in desire for some women. To date, there are no FDA-approved medications for the treatment of low desire in postmenopausal women.

Appendix B

MEN'S SEXUAL AROUSAL

"The relationship between a man and his penis is profound and consequential" (Watter, 2023, p. 12). We do a disservice to men when we doubt the veracity of this statement. All too often, in an attempt to control how he is viewed by others and how he is perceived by a partner he desires or loves (or both), a man will try to control the behavior of his penis. This is usually a failing strategy, because the penis responds, not to anxious commands, but to erotic and desired stimulation. The penis can also be a "conduit for male emotion," regulating "the closeness and distance that men will allow themselves to experience in intimate relationships" (Watter, 2023, p. 14). The penis is a remarkable organ, and its response to erotic stimulation will be described in some detail in the following paragraphs. Unless otherwise stated, the anatomical and physiological information about penile functioning comes from Levay and Valente's (2006) textbook on human sexuality.

SIZE

Given the importance of the penis, it is no wonder that men are highly anxious about how it functions and how it looks. In terms of appearance, size seems to be the main concern. Most men believe that the average length of the penis is over 6 inches (when erect). In fact, the average length of an erect penis hovers somewhere around 5.1 inches (and maybe less, given the likelihood of volunteer bias—men with smaller penises may not want to participate in a study measuring penile length; Veale et al., 2015). This means that there are many men with perfectly average sized penises thinking that they are inadequate and small. And this matters, because how a man relates to his penis is important for his sexual pleasure.

ANATOMY

The penis is comprised of the shaft and the head or glans at the top of the shaft. Atop the head of the penis is the *meatus*, or the opening through which sperm or urine is expelled (but thanks to the urethral sphincter, not at the same time). The glans has a rim, called the *corona*, which encircles the penis. On the underside of the penis, where the corona is shaped like an inverted V and almost meets the tip of the glans, there is a loose strip of skin called the *frenulum*. The corona and the frenulum are the most sexually sensitive areas of the penis, and stimulation in this area is usually highly erotic. At the base of the penis sits the scrotum or scrotal sac, which holds the testicles.

ERECTION

When a man is sexually aroused, the brain signals for the release of neurotransmitters necessary to start the process of vasodilation (blood flow to the penis). Inside the shaft of the penis are two cylindrical structures called the *corpora cavernosa*, which are filled with spongelike tissue. These structures fill with blood, expanding the erectile tissue and cutting off blood flow, so not only does blood no longer flow in, but also it does not flow out. Thus, the penis is erect and stays erect if arousal is maintained.

With rising levels of sexual arousal, there is an increase in sympathetic nervous system activity, including rapid breathing and increased heart rate and blood pressure. Muscle contractions cause further swelling of the penis, and the testicles are drawn upward, sometimes to the point of disappearing from view. When arousal reaches a certain point, the process is reversed—and orgasm reflexively occurs.

EJACULATION AND ORGASM

Contrary to popular belief, a man can ejaculate with a flaccid penis. The physiology of ejaculation and the physiology of erection are different, even though both require sexual arousal. As sexual arousal increases (whether or not the penis is erect), semen is released into the posterior portion of the urethra. Men will often feel a pulsing sensation at the base of the penis during this time. This is the point of ejaculatory inevitability, where it is virtually impossible for a man to avoid ejaculation. Spasmodic contractions of the smooth muscles of the pelvic floor and the smooth muscle in the walls of the urethra combine to forcefully expel the semen. This is ejaculation.

TIMING OF EJACULATION

The median time for ejaculation during heterosexual intercourse is a little over 5 minutes, as reported in a study where men timed themselves using stopwatches (Waldinger et al., 2005). Premature ejaculation (PE) is defined as ejaculation that occurs too quickly (usually less than 2 minutes) during penile–vaginal intercourse or other sexual stimulation. Men enjoy prolonging pleasurable sexual experiences, and they like to feel in control of when they ejaculate (within reason). A consult with a sex therapist or sexual medicine specialist should be considered when men complain of PE.

Edging is the practice of getting aroused and then pulling back just prior to ejaculatory inevitability, and doing this several times, to prolong the sexual experience at a high level of arousal. Some men also believe that edging increases the pleasurable sensations of their orgasm.

REFRACTORY PERIOD

Men have a refractory period, a variable length of time following ejaculation during which they are unable to be stimulated to achieve an erection or orgasm. The length of the refractory period varies with age, health, and stimulation. A novel and desirable sex partner, for example, can shorten the refractory period for most men. The refractory period is longer for older men, and many older men (60 plus) may choose to enjoy sex more frequently by (purposefully) not ejaculating with every sexual encounter.

Appendix C

SENSATE FOCUS INSTRUCTIONS FOR CLIENTS

Sensate focus is one of the mainstays of behavioral sex therapy. It is often used early in the treatment of most, if not all, sexual dysfunctions. While sensate focus has been reimagined and reinterpreted by sex therapists over time, these instructions follow Masters and Johnson's original intention. This is a lightly edited reprint of a handout Linda Weiner, LCSW, gives to her patients.[1] Weiner is an advocate of the traditional Masters and Johnson approach to mindful touch and coauthor of the illustrated manual of sensate focus (Weiner & Avery-Clark, 2017).

PURPOSE OF SENSATE FOCUS

Sensate focus mindful touch forms the basis of sex therapy, as it teaches a strategy for lowering anxiety, turning off the mind, and reinhabiting the body—all essential for developing sexual interest and response.

The goal of sensate focus is not to experience turn-on, erotic feelings, or even, necessarily, feelings of pleasure. One purpose is to learn about one's own bodily responses and feelings, whatever they are. A second purpose is to learn to tune into the body by focusing on bodily sensations and to mindfully bring attention back to the body when the mind is active with distractions. Another purpose is to learn that touching can be as intimate (or more so) as intercourse or penetrative sex and is a good end in and of itself, aiding couples to feel close and connected. Still another purpose is for the couple to experience that erotic feelings may eventually arise from touch without pressure.

[1] Appendix C is from *Sensate Focus Instructions for Clients* [Handout], by L. Weiner (personal communication, January 8, 2025). Copyright 2025 by Linda Weiner (https://www.sextherapiststlouis.com/). Reprinted with permission.

INSTRUCTIONS FOR SENSATE FOCUS

No intercourse, oral sex, or mutual masturbation is suggested during this experience or immediately thereafter. The reason it works is that there is no pressure to want it, like it, or have to respond in any particular way.

Arrange for one hour of complete privacy when you are not exhausted. Relax together first, then each touches the partner (with hands and fingers) front to back and top to bottom, avoiding breast and genital touching at first, for 5–15 minutes, then switch. Eventually, when you are able to touch for self (i.e., touching one's partner for your own interest), focus on sensations, and bring yourself back from distractions, breasts and genitals are added as any other part of the body (no "camping out"; in other words, don't linger too long on the breasts and genitals). You can flip a coin to see who goes first.

Alcohol or recreational drugs are not recommended.

Set the mood for relaxation by sitting on the couch together, sharing a meal, etc. Instrumental music and low lighting are fine.

Temperature should be arranged for comfort ahead of time.

Touching experiences should be scheduled 1–3 times per week, and usually two will happen! Let your partner know when you plan to do the touching, or schedule it on a calendar.

Clothing off as much as possible, some lighting on, pets elsewhere, door secured.

Using hands and fingers only, focus your attention on the sensations of temperature (warm or cool), texture of hair and skin (smooth or rough), and pressure (firm or soft) as you touch your partner for YOUR INTEREST, not his or her pleasure. This is not a massage, which is for the OTHER. This is often the most challenging part as most of us were taught that touch is for the partner's pleasure.

Kissing and full body contact are not recommended.

Try not to talk to each other, though the initial discomfort may induce you to talk, giggle, or feel ticklish.

Protect your partner from doing anything physically or psychologically UNCOMFORTABLE by moving their hand away for now. The partner is then free to touch any way they wish without concern for how things are going for you, as you will let them know!

Notice the following:

Temperature: Where are you and your partner warmer or cooler? Does that change?

Texture: Of hair and skin. Where are they smoother? Rougher? What are the textures?

Pressure: How does it feel to me when I use or experience a firmer or lighter touch?

TOUCHER

It is important to:

Experiment with positioning one's body to find a comfortable way of touching your partner.

Initiate by saying, "I'd like to touch now." Touchee can decline, but if they do, they are responsible for reinitiating.

Focus on one's own feelings without judgment, whether touching or being touched.

Be concerned with one's own experience and sensations rather than with the partner (e.g., wondering if he/she is bored, tired, turned on or off). Trust that your partner will protect you from doing anything psychologically or physically uncomfortable by communicating that to you, nonverbally if possible.

If your mind wanders, bring it back to temperature, texture, pressure. If it continues to wander, decide how to manage it or stop.

Touch long enough to get over any initial feelings of discomfort, but not so long as to get tired or bored (5–15 minutes usually does it).

TOUCHEE

The touchee is to get as comfortable as possible. You may begin in any position, such as your stomach, and move to other positions as you wish.

The touchee is encouraged to focus on his/her sensations coming in through the fingertips (whatever they are) and not to be concerned with what his/her partner is experiencing. Bring yourself back from distractions and protect your partner by letting him/her know, nonverbally if possible, if something is psychologically or physically uncomfortable.

If your mind wanders, refocus on temperature, texture, or pressure. If it continues to wander, decide how to manage it or stop. Touch long enough to get over any initial feelings of discomfort, but not so long as to get tired or bored (5–15 minutes usually does it).

COUPLE

Following the touching, lie together for a bit, then write down something about the experience of touching for self, focusing on sensations, [and noticing] any distractions and how you handled them and bring this information to your next session. At the early stage, couples do not yet have the skills to talk about the touching without evaluating how it went.

As you become more adept, breasts and genitals as well as mutual touching and genital-to-genital contact will be added. Also, in Stage 2, when the sexual difficulty has been resolved, you will be encouraged to share what you like. But this is the foundation!

Appendix D

RESOURCES

PROFESSIONAL SOCIETIES: SEXUAL MEDICINE

Each of these websites has a "Find a Provider" tab so you can locate a sexual medicine specialist in your area. They also have resources for patients that contain helpful information on various conditions. These resources are helpful for clinicians too.

Herman & Wallace Pelvic Rehabilitation Institute: https://hermanwallace.com/
International Society for the Scientific Study of Women's Sexual Health (ISSWSH): https://www.isswsh.org/
International Society for Sexual Medicine (ISSM): https://www.issm.info/
North American Menopause Society (NAMS): https://www.menopause.org/
Sexual Medicine Society of North America (SMSNA): https://www.smsna.org/

PROFESSIONAL SOCIETIES: SEX THERAPY

Each of these websites has a "Find a Provider" tab so you can locate a sex therapist in your area. They also list conferences and continuing education opportunities.

American Association of Sexuality Educators, Counselors and Therapists (AASECT): https://www.aasect.org/
Kinsey Institute: https://kinseyinstitute.org/
The Kinsey Institute website contains valuable resources, links to educational and professional meetings, and access to some of their collections of articles and books.
Society for Sex Therapy and Research (SSTAR): https://sstarnet.org/

ONLINE RESOURCES FOR PATIENTS

OMG.YES: https://www.omgyes.com/
This website provides information and techniques regarding sexual stimulation for individuals and/or couples, complete with videos and animations to illustrate. A one-time fee is assessed for users.

Sex Smart Films: https://sexsmartfilms.com/
This resource provides access to a library of sex education, sex therapy, and sex research films, including demonstrations of sensate focus for heterosexual, gay, and lesbian couples. Some films are dated, while others are quite current.

BOOKS FOR PROFESSIONALS: SEX THERAPY

Buehler, S. (2021). *What every mental health professional needs to know about sex* (3rd ed.). Springer Publishing.
This clearly written book is a great starting point for those interested in learning more about sex therapy techniques for the treatment of sexual dysfunctions.

Goerlich, S. (2020). *The leather couch*. Routledge.
This is an invaluable resource for ethically and effectively providing therapy to members of the kink community.

Goerlich, S. (2022). *Kink-affirming practice: Culturally competent therapy from the leather chair*. Routledge.
Another invaluable resource for ethically and effectively providing therapy to members of the kink community.

Hall, K. S. K., & Binik, Y. M. (2020). *Principles and practice of sex therapy* (6th ed.). The Guilford Press.
This is a more advanced text that integrates relevant research with state-of-the-art therapy for sexual dysfunctions and sexual problems.

Watter, D. N. (2023). *The existential importance of the penis: A guide to understanding male sexuality*. Routledge.
This is one of the few books on male sexuality. It takes a compassionate approach to understanding the distress many men face when confronted with sexual problems. The book is fascinating to read and clinically invaluable.

Weiner, L., & Avery-Clark, C. (2017). *Sensate focus in sex therapy: The illustrated manual*. Routledge.
This step-by-step guide to sensate focus is the way Masters and Johnson intended it. This book is a great starting guide to have if you intend to use sensate focus with patients. The illustrations are helpful and tasteful.

GENERAL SEX INFORMATION FOR PATIENTS AND CLINICIANS

Brotto, L. A. (2018). *Better sex through mindfulness: How women can cultivate desire*. Greystone Books.

This illustrated book is a compassionate guide to using mindfulness techniques for women who want to experience greater levels of sexual pleasure and desire.

Joannides, P. (2022). *The guide to getting it on: Unzipped* (10th ed.). Goofy Foot Press.

Hands down, this work is the most comprehensive and accurate sex book on the market. This well-researched and clearly written book will appeal to adult patients of all ages. It is written with humor and illustrated by the comic book artist Dærick Gröss Sr.

References

Abramson, P. R., Mosher, D. L., Abramson, L. M., & Wotchowski, B. (1977). Personality correlates of the Mosher Guilt Scales. *Journal of Personality Assessment, 41*(4), 375–382. https://doi.org/10.1207/s15327752jpa4104_7

Abu-Raya, N. E., & Gewirtz-Meydan, A. (2023). Childhood sexual abuse and relationship satisfaction: The moderating role of PTSD and sexual-related posttraumatic stress symptoms. *Journal of Sex & Marital Therapy, 49*(8), 996–1012. https://doi.org/10.1080/0092623X.2023.2237510

Agochukwu-Mmonu, N., Malani, P. N., Wittmann, D., Kirch, M., Kullgren, J., Singer, D., & Solway, E. (2021). Interest in sex and conversations about sexual health with health care providers among older U.S. adults. *Clinical Gerontologist, 44*(3), 299–306. https://doi.org/10.1080/07317115.2021.1882637

American Association of Sex Educators, Counselors and Therapists. (n.d.). *AASECT requirements for sex therapy certification*. https://www.aasect.org/aasect-requirements-sex-therapist-certification

American Psychiatric Association. (1980). *Diagnostic and statistical manual of mental disorders* (3rd ed.).

American Psychiatric Association. (1987). *Diagnostic and statistical manual of mental disorders* (3rd ed., rev.).

American Psychiatric Association. (2013). *Diagnostic and statistical manual of mental disorders* (5th ed.). https://doi.org/10.1176/appi.books.9780890425596

American Psychiatric Association. (2022). *Diagnostic and statistical manual of mental disorders* (5th ed., text rev.). https://doi.org/10.1176/appi.books.9780890425787

American Psychological Association. (2022). *Resolution on appropriate affirmative responses to sexual orientation distress and change efforts*. https://www.apa.org/about/policy/sexual-orientation

Amphis, Marnanel, & Xeror. (2017, August 21). *Internal anatomy of the human vulva, focusing on the anatomy and location of the clitoris* [Figure]. Wikimedia Commons. https://commons.wikimedia.org/wiki/File:Clitoris_Anatomy.svg

Angier, N. (2000). *Woman: An intimate geography*. Anchor Books.

Anzani, A., Lindley, L., Tognasso, G., Galupo, M. P., & Prunas, A. (2021). "Being talked to like I was a sex toy, like being transgender was simply for the enjoyment of someone else": Fetishization and sexualization of transgender and non-binary individuals. *Archives of Sexual Behavior*, *50*(3), 897–911. https://doi.org/10.1007/s10508-021-01935-8

Argenti Aertheri. (2023, August 11). *Sexual response cycle as first described by Masters and Johnson* [Figure]. Wikimedia Commons. https://commons.wikimedia.org/wiki/File:Sexual-response-cycle.svg

Bailey, T. D., & Brown, L. S. (2021). Treating clients who have been sexually abused by a therapist. In A. Steinberg, J. L. Alpert, & C. A. Courtois (Eds.), *Sexual boundary violations in psychotherapy: Facing therapist indiscretions, transgressions, and misconduct* (pp. 319–341). American Psychological Association. https://doi.org/10.1037/0000247-018

Bancroft, J., & Janssen, E. (2000). The dual control model of male sexual response: A theoretical approach to centrally mediated erectile dysfunction. *Neuroscience and Biobehavioral Reviews*, *24*(5), 571–579. https://doi.org/10.1016/S0149-7634(00)00024-5

Bancroft, J., Janssen, E., Strong, D., & Vukadinovic, Z. (2003). The relation between mood and sexuality in gay men. *Archives of Sexual Behavior*, *32*(3), 231–242. https://doi.org/10.1023/A:1023461500810

Bártová, K., Androvičová, R., Krejčová, L., Weiss, P., & Klapilová, K. (2021). The prevalence of paraphilic interests in the Czech population: Preference, arousal, the use of pornography, fantasy, and behavior. *Journal of Sex Research*, *58*(1), 86–96. https://doi.org/10.1080/00224499.2019.1707468

Basson, R. (2001). Human sex-response cycles. *Journal of Sex & Marital Therapy*, *27*(1), 33–43. https://doi.org/10.1080/00926230152035831

Beach, F. A. (1956). Characteristics of masculine "sex drive." In M. R. Jones (Ed.), *Nebraska symposium on motivation* (pp. 1–32). University of Nebraska Press.

Benjamin, L. T., Jr., Whitaker, J. L., Ramsey, R. M., & Zeve, D. R. (2007). John B. Watson's alleged sex research: An appraisal of the evidence. *American Psychologist*, *62*(2), 131–139. https://doi.org/10.1037/0003-066X.62.2.131

Bergner, D. (2009, January 22). What do women want? *New York Times Magazine*. https://www.nytimes.com/2009/01/25/magazine/25desire-t.html

Bigras, N., Vaillancourt-Morel, M. P., Nolin, M. C., & Bergeron, S. (2021). Associations between childhood sexual abuse and sexual well-being in adulthood: A systematic literature review. *Journal of Child Sexual Abuse*, *30*(3), 332–352. https://doi.org/10.1080/10538712.2020.1825148

Bonagura, A., Abrams, D., & Teller, J. (2022). Diagnostic differential between pedophilic-OCD and pedophilic disorder: An illustration with two vignettes. *Archives of Sexual Behavior*, *51*(4), 2359–2368. https://doi.org/10.1007/s10508-021-02273-5

Bőthe, B., Nagy, L., Koós, M., Demetrovics, Z., Potenza, M. N., Kraus, S. W., & International Sex Survey Consortium. (2024). Problematic pornography use across countries, genders, and sexual orientations: Insights from the International

Sex Survey and comparison of different assessment tools. *Addiction, 119*(5), 928–950. https://doi.org/10.1111/add.16431

Bőthe, B., Tóth-Király, I., Demetrovics, Z., & Orosz, G. (2021). The short version of the Problematic Pornography Consumption Scale (PPCS-6): A reliable and valid measure in general and treatment-seeking populations. *Journal of Sex Research, 58*(3), 342–352. https://doi.org/10.1080/00224499.2020.1716205

Bőthe, B., Tóth-Király, I., Zsila, Á., Griffiths, M. D., Demetrovics, Z., & Orosz, G. (2018). The development of the Problematic Pornography Consumption Scale (PPCS). *Journal of Sex Research, 55*(3), 395–406. https://doi.org/10.1080/00224499.2017.1291798

Bőthe, B., Vaillancourt-Morel, M. P., & Bergeron, S. (2022). Associations between pornography use frequency, pornography use motivations, and sexual well-being in couples. *Journal of Sex Research, 59*(4), 457–471. https://doi.org/10.1080/00224499.2021.1893261

Bőthe, B., Vaillancourt-Morel, M. P., Bergeron, S., Hermann, Z., Ivaskevics, K., Kraus, S. W., Grubbs, J. B., & the Problematic Pornography Use Machine Learning Study Consortium. (2024). Uncovering the most robust predictors of problematic pornography use: A large-scale machine learning study across 16 countries. *Journal of Psychopathology and Clinical Science, 133*(6), 489–502. Advance online publication. https://doi.org/10.1037/abn0000913

Brecher, E. M. (1969). *The sex researchers*. Little, Brown and Company.

Briere, J. (1996). A self-trauma model for treating adult survivors of severe child abuse. In J. Briere, L. Berliner, J. A. Bulkley, C. Jenny, & T. Reid (Eds.), *The APSAC handbook on child maltreatment* (pp. 140–157). SAGE Publications.

Bronski, M. (2004). Foreword. In P. Moore (Ed.), *Beyond shame: Reclaiming the abandoned history of radical gay sexuality* (pp. xiii–xx). Beacon Press.

Brotto, L. A., & Yule, M. (2017). Asexuality: Sexual orientation, paraphilia, sexual dysfunction, or none of the above? *Archives of Sexual Behavior, 46*(3), 619–627. https://doi.org/10.1007/s10508-016-0802-7

Brown, V., Haffner, G., Holmstrand, D., Oakum, C., Orbuch, E., Pavlock, V., & Pepperl, S. (2020). Rape and sexual assault. *The Georgetown Journal of Gender and the Law, 21*, 367–392.

Bruce, S. L., Ching, T. H. W., & Williams, M. T. (2018). Pedophilia-themed obsessive–compulsive disorder: Assessment, differential diagnosis, and treatment with exposure and response prevention. *Archives of Sexual Behavior, 47*(2), 389–402. https://doi.org/10.1007/s10508-017-1031-4

Campbell, C., Scoats, R., & Wignall, L. (2023). "Oh! How modern! And . . . are you OK with that?": Consensually non-monogamous people's experiences when accessing sexual health care. *Journal of Sex Research, 61*(9), 1377–1388. https://doi.org/10.1080/00224499.2023.2246464

Cantor, J. M. (2014). "Gold-star pedophiles" in general sex therapy practice. In Y. M. Binik & K. S. K. Hall (Eds.), *Principles and practice of sex therapy* (5th ed., pp. 219–234). The Guilford Press.

Carson, S. A., & Kallen, A. N. (2021). Diagnosis and management of infertility: A review. *JAMA, 326*(1), 65–76. https://doi.org/10.1001/jama.2021.4788

Caruso, S., Palermo, G., Caruso, G., & Rapisarda, A. M. C. (2022). How does contraceptive use affect women's sexuality? A novel look at sexual acceptability. *Journal of Clinical Medicine, 11*(3), 810–820. https://doi.org/10.3390/jcm11030810

Cass, V. (2004). *The elusive orgasm: A woman's guide to why she can't and how she can orgasm*. Brightfire.

Cheeseborough, T., Overstreet, N., & Ward, L. M. (2020). Interpersonal sexual objectification, Jezebel stereotype endorsement, and justification of intimate partner violence toward women. *Psychology of Women Quarterly, 44*(2), 203–216. https://doi.org/10.1177/0361684319896345

Chen, Y.-L., Huang, K.-J., Scoglio, A. A. J., Borgogna, N. C., Potenza, M. N., Blycker, G. R., & Kraus, S. W. (2024). A network comparison of sexual dysfunction, psychological factors, and body dissociation between individuals with and without sexual trauma histories. *Journal of Trauma & Dissociation, 25*(1), 62–82. https://doi.org/10.1080/15299732.2023.2231915

Christina, G. (2023). Are we having sex now or what? In R. Halwani, J. M. Held, N. McKeever, & A. Soble (Eds.), *The philosophy of sex* (8th ed., pp. 15–21). Rowman & Littlefield.

Conley, T. D., Matsick, J. L., Moors, A. C., Ziegler, A., & Rubin, J. D. (2015). Re-examining the effectiveness of monogamy as an STI-preventive strategy. *Preventive Medicine, 78*, 23–28. https://doi.org/10.1016/j.ypmed.2015.06.006

Cruz, C., Greenwald, E., & Sandil, R. (2017). Let's talk about sex: Integrating sex positivity in counseling psychology practice. *The Counseling Psychologist, 45*(4), 547–569. https://doi.org/10.1177/0011000017714763

Curtiz, M. (Director). (1942). Casablanca [Film]. Warner Bros.

Demant, D., Byron, P., Oviedo-Trespalacios, O., Saliba, B., & Newton, J. D. (2024). The nexus between porn and psychosocial/psychosexual well-being among gay and bisexual men. *Porn Studies*, 1–17. https://doi.org/10.1080/23268743.2024.2335975

Dyer, K., & das Nair, R. (2013). Why don't healthcare professionals talk about sex? A systematic review of recent qualitative studies conducted in the United Kingdom. *Journal of Sexual Medicine, 10*(11), 2658–2670. https://doi.org/10.1111/j.1743-6109.2012.02856.x

Easton, S. D., Saltzman, L. Y., & Willis, D. G. (2014). "Would you tell under circumstances like that?": Barriers to disclosure of child sexual abuse for men. *Psychology of Men & Masculinities, 15*(4), 460–469. https://doi.org/10.1037/a0034223

Elise, D. (2008). Sex and shame: The inhibition of female desires. *Journal of the American Psychoanalytic Association, 56*(1), 73–98. https://doi.org/10.1177/0003065108315685

Emmers-Sommer, T. M., Allen, M., Vadona Schoenbauer, K., & Burrell, N. (2018). Implications of sex guilt: A meta-analysis. *Marriage & Family Review, 54*(5), 417–437. https://doi.org/10.1080/01494929.2017.1359815

Emond, M., Byers, E. S., Brassard, A., Tremblay, N., & Péloquin, K. (2024). Addressing sexual issues in couples seeking relationship therapy. *Sexual and Relationship Therapy*, *39*(1), 115–130. https://doi.org/10.1080/14681994.2021.1969546

Farber, B. A., Blanchard, M., & Love, M. (2019). *Secrets and lies in psychotherapy*. American Psychological Association. https://doi.org/10.1037/0000128-000

Fern, J. (2020). *Polysecure: Attachment, trauma and consensual nonmonogamy*. Thorntree Press.

Fernet, M., Hébert, M., Brodeur, G., & Théorêt, V. (2021). "When you're in a relationship, you say no, but your partner insists": Sexual dating violence and ambiguity among girls and young women. *Journal of Interpersonal Violence*, *36*(19–20), 9436–9459. https://doi.org/10.1177/0886260519867149

Fife, S. T., Gossner, J. D., Theobald, A., Allen, E., Rivero, A., & Koehl, H. (2023). Couple healing from infidelity: A grounded theory study. *Journal of Social and Personal Relationships*, *40*(12), 3882–3905. https://doi.org/10.1177/02654075231177874

Finkelhor, D. (1990). Early and long-term effects of child sexual abuse: An update. *Professional Psychology: Research and Practice*, *21*(5), 325–330. https://doi.org/10.1037/0735-7028.21.5.325

Finkelhor, D., & Browne, A. (1985). The traumatic impact of child sexual abuse: A conceptualization. *American Journal of Orthopsychiatry*, *55*(4), 530–541. https://doi.org/10.1111/j.1939-0025.1985.tb02703.x

Fischer, N., & Træen, B. (2022). A seemingly paradoxical relationship between masturbation frequency and sexual satisfaction. *Archives of Sexual Behavior*, *51*, 3151–3167. https://doi.org/10.1007/s10508-022-02305-8

Fortenberry, J. D., & Hensel, D. J. (2022). Sexual modesty in sexual expression and experience: A scoping review, 2000–2021. *Journal of Sex Research*, *59*(8), 1000–1014. https://doi.org/10.1080/00224499.2021.2016571

Fox, M. H., Seto, M. C., Refaie, N., Lavrinsek, S., Hall, V., Curry, S., Ashbaugh, A. R., Levaque, E., Fedoroff, J. P., Bradford, J. M., & Lalumière, M. L. (2022). The relation between the paraphilias and anxiety in men: A case–control study. *Archives of Sexual Behavior*, *51*(8), 4063–4084. https://doi.org/10.1007/s10508-022-02346-z

Frederick, D. A., Gillespie, B. J., Lever, J., Berardi, V., & Garcia, J. R. (2021). Debunking lesbian bed death: Using coarsened exact matching to compare sexual practices and satisfaction of lesbian and heterosexual women. *Archives of Sexual Behavior*, *50*(8), 3601–3619. https://doi.org/10.1007/s10508-021-02096-4

Freud, S. (1905). Three essays on the theory of sexuality. In J. Strachey & A. Freud (Eds.), *The standard edition of the complete works of Sigmund Freud: Vol. 7. A case of hysteria, three essays on sexuality and other works, 1901–1905* (pp. 123–246). Hogarth Press.

Friday, N. (1973). *My secret garden: Women's sexual fantasies*. Rosetta Books.

Friday, N. (1980). *Men in love*. Rosetta Books.

Gewirtz, P. (1996). On "I know it when I see it." *The Yale Law Journal, 105*(4), 1023–1047. https://doi.org/10.2307/797245

Gewirtz-Meydan, A., & Lassri, D. (2023). Sex in the shadow of child sexual abuse: The development and psychometric evaluation of the post-traumatic sexuality (PT-SEX) scale. *Journal of Interpersonal Violence, 38*(5–6), 4714–4741. https://doi.org/10.1177/08862605221118969

Gewirtz-Meydan, A., & Opuda, E. (2022). The impact of child sexual abuse on men's sexual function: A systematic review. *Trauma, Violence, & Abuse, 23*(1), 265–277. https://doi.org/10.1177/1524838020939134

Gewirtz-Meydan, A., & Opuda, E. (2023). The sexual fantasies of childhood sexual abuse survivors: A rapid review. *Trauma, Violence, & Abuse, 24*(2), 441–453. https://doi.org/10.1177/15248380211030487

Goren, E. (2021). The art of helpful sex talk in therapy: A psychoanalytic sex therapist speaks. In A. Steinberg, J. L. Alpert, & C. A. Courtois (Eds.), *Sexual boundary violations in psychotherapy: Facing therapist indiscretions, transgressions, and misconduct* (pp. 129–139). American Psychological Association. https://doi.org/10.1037/0000247-008

Graham, C. A., Sanders, S. A., & Milhausen, R. R. (2006). The sexual excitation/sexual inhibition inventory for women: Psychometric properties. *Archives of Sexual Behavior, 35*(4), 397–409. https://doi.org/10.1007/s10508-006-9041-7

Graham, C. A., Sanders, S. A., Milhausen, R. R., & McBride, K. R. (2004). Turning on and turning off: A focus group study of the factors that affect women's sexual arousal. *Archives of Sexual Behavior, 33*(6), 527–538. https://doi.org/10.1023/B:ASEB.0000044737.62561.fd

Griffiths, M. (2005). A "components" model of addiction within a biopsychosocial framework. *Journal of Substance Use, 10*(4), 191–197. https://doi.org/10.1080/14659890500114359

Grubbs, J. B., Floyd, C. G., Griffin, K. R., Jennings, T. L., & Kraus, S. W. (2022). Moral incongruence and addiction: A registered report. *Psychology of Addictive Behaviors, 36*(7), 749–761. https://doi.org/10.1037/adb0000876

Gupta, S., Tarantino, M., & Sanner, C. (2024). A scoping review of research on polyamory and consensual non-monogamy: Implications for a more inclusive family science. *Journal of Family Theory & Review, 16*(2), 151–190. https://doi.org/10.1111/jftr.12546

Hall, K. S. K. (2019). Cultural differences in the treatment of sex problems. *Current Sexual Health Reports, 11*(1), 29–34. https://doi.org/10.1007/s11930-019-00189-9

Hall, K. S. K., & Graham, C. A. (Eds.). (2012). *The cultural context of sexual pleasure and problems: Psychotherapy with diverse clients*. Routledge. https://doi.org/10.4324/9780203096833

Hall, K. S. K., & Graham, C. A. (2014). Culturally sensitive sex therapy. In Y. M. Binik & K. S. K. Hall (Eds.), *Principles and practice of sex therapy* (5th ed., pp. 334–358). The Guilford Press.

Hall, K. S. K., & Graham, C. A. (2020). The privileging of pleasure. In K. S. K. Hall & Y. M. Binik (Eds.), *Principles and practice of sex therapy* (6th ed., pp. 243–268). The Guilford Press.

Harris, E. A., Hornsey, M. J., Hofmann, W., Jern, P., Murphy, S. C., Hedenborg, F., & Barlow, F. K. (2023). Does sexual desire fluctuate more among women than men? *Archives of Sexual Behavior, 52*(4), 1461–1478. https://doi.org/10.1007/s10508-022-02525-y

Heiman, J. R., Long, J. S., Smith, S. N., Fisher, W. A., Sand, M. S., & Rosen, R. C. (2011). Sexual satisfaction and relationship happiness in midlife and older couples in five countries. *Archives of Sexual Behavior, 40*(4), 741–753. https://doi.org/10.1007/s10508-010-9703-3

Herbenick, D., Bowling, J., Fu, T.-C., Dodge, B., Guerra-Reyes, L., & Sanders, S. (2017). Sexual diversity in the United States: Results from a nationally representative probability sample of adult women and men. *PLOS ONE, 12*(7), e0181198. https://doi.org/10.1371/journal.pone.0181198

Herbenick, D., Eastman-Mueller, H., Fu, T.-C., Dodge, B., Ponander, K., & Sanders, S. A. (2019). Women's sexual satisfaction, communication, and reasons for (no longer) faking orgasm: Findings from a U.S. probability sample. *Archives of Sexual Behavior, 48*, 2461–2472. https://doi.org/10.1007/s10508-019-01493-0

Herbenick, D., Fu, T.-C., & Patterson, C. (2023). Sexual repertoire, duration of partnered sex, sexual pleasure, and orgasm: Findings from a US nationally representative survey of adults. *Journal of Sex & Marital Therapy, 49*(4), 369–390. https://doi.org/10.1080/0092623X.2022.2126417

Herbenick, D., Fu, T.-C., Arter, J., Sanders, S. A., & Dodge, B. (2018). Women's experiences with genital touching, sexual pleasure, and orgasm: Results from a US probability sample of women ages 18 to 94. *Journal of Sex & Marital Therapy, 44*(2), 201–212. https://doi.org/10.1080/0092623X.2017.1346530

Hermann, L., Baba, A., Montagner, D., Parker, R., Smiga, J. A., Tomaskovic-Moore, S., Walfrand, A., Miller, T. L., Weis, R., Bauer, C., Campos, A., Jackson, E., Johnston, M., Khan, S., Lutz, G. D., Nguyen, H., & Niederhoff, T. (2020). *2020 Ace Community Survey summary report*. https://acecommunitysurvey.org/2022/10/27/2020-ace-community-survey-summary-report/

Hiemstra, J., van Tuijl, P., & van Lankveld, J. (2024). The associations of sexual desire, daily stress, and intimacy in gay men in long-term relationships. *International Journal of Impotence Research, 36*(3), 248–255. https://doi.org/10.1038/s41443-023-00664-x

Hille, J. J., Simmons, M. K., & Sanders, S. A. (2020). "Sex" and the ace spectrum: Definitions of sex, behavioral histories, and future interest for individuals who identify as asexual, graysexual, or demisexual. *Journal of Sex Research, 57*(7), 813–823. https://doi.org/10.1080/00224499.2019.1689378

Holvoet, L., Huys, W., Coppens, V., Seeuws, J., Goethals, K., & Morrens, M. (2017). Fifty shades of Belgian gray: The prevalence of BDSM-related fantasies and activities in the general population. *Journal of Sexual Medicine, 14*(9), 1152–1159. https://doi.org/10.1016/J.JSXM.2017.07.003

Hook, J. N., Farrell, J. E., Davis, D. E., DeBlaere, C., Van Tongeren, D. R., & Utsey, S. O. (2016). Cultural humility and racial microaggressions in counseling. *Journal of Counseling Psychology, 63*(3), 269–277. https://doi.org/10.1037/cou0000114

Hui, A., Salkovskis, P., & Rumble-Browne, J. (2024). The impact of childhood sexual abuse on interpersonal violence in men: A systematic review. *Aggression and Violent Behavior, 78*, 101928. Advance online publication. https://doi.org/10.1016/j.avb.2024.101928

Huntington, C., Markman, H., & Rhoades, G. (2021). Watching pornography alone or together: Longitudinal associations with romantic relationship quality. *Journal of Sex & Marital Therapy, 47*(2), 130–146. https://doi.org/10.1080/0092623X.2020.1835760

Jeffrey, N. K., & Barata, P. C. (2021). Intimate partner sexual violence among Canadian university students: Incidence, context, and perpetrators' perceptions. *Archives of Sexual Behavior, 50*(5), 2123–2138. https://doi.org/10.1007/s10508-021-02006-8

Jong, E. (1973). *Fear of flying*. Penguin Books.

Josephs, L. (2018). *The dynamics of infidelity: Applying relationship science to psychotherapy practice*. American Psychological Association. https://doi.org/10.1037/0000053-000

Josephs, L. (2020). Restoring trust and sexual intimacy after infidelities. In K. S. K. Hall & Y. M. Binik (Eds.), *Principles and practices of sex therapy* (6th ed., pp. 317–330). The Guilford Press.

Joyal, C. C. (2021). Problems and controversies with psychiatric diagnoses of paraphilia. In L. A. Craig & R. M. Bartels (Eds.), *Sexual deviance: Understanding and managing deviant sexual interests and paraphilic disorders* (pp. 91–116). Wiley Blackwell. https://doi.org/10.1002/9781119771401.ch6

Joyal, C. C., & Carpentier, J. (2017). The prevalence of paraphilic interests and behaviors in the general population: A provincial survey. *Journal of Sex Research, 54*(2), 161–171. https://doi.org/10.1080/00224499.2016.1139034

Joyal, C. C., Cossette, A., & Lapierre, V. (2015). What exactly is an unusual sexual fantasy? *Journal of Sexual Medicine, 12*(2), 328–340. https://doi.org/10.1111/jsm.12734

Kaplan, H. S. (1974). *The new sex therapy*. Brunner/Mazel.

Keilholtz, B. M., & Spencer, C. M. (2022). Couples therapy and intimate partner violence: Considerations, assessment, and treatment modalities. *Practice Innovations, 7*(2), 124–137. https://doi.org/10.1037/pri0000176

Khani, S., Azizi, M., Elyasi, F., Kamali, M., & Moosazadeh, M. (2021). The prevalence of sexual dysfunction in the different menopausal stages: A systematic review and meta-analysis. *International Journal of Sexual Health, 33*(3), 439–472. https://doi.org/10.1080/19317611.2021.1926039

Kinsey, A. C., Pomeroy, W. B., Martin, C. E., & Gebhard, P. H. (1948). *Sexual behavior in the human male*. Indiana University Press.

Kinsey, A. C., Pomeroy, W. B., Martin, C. E., & Gebhard, P. H. (1953). *Sexual behavior in the human female*. Indiana University Press.

Koós, M., Nagy, L., Kraus, S. W., Demetrovics, Z., Potenza, M. N., Gaudet, É., Ballester-Arnal, R., Batthyány, D., Bergeron, S., Billieux, J., Briken, P., Burkauskas, J., Cárdenas-López, G., Carvalho, J., Castro-Calvo, J., Chang, Y.-H., Chen, L., Ciocca, G., Corazza, O., . . . Bőthe, B. (2024). Why do people watch pornography? Cross-cultural validation of the Pornography Use Motivations Scale (PUMS) and its short form (PUMS-8). *Journal of Sex Research, 62*(6), 1049–1065. https://doi.org/10.1080/00224499.2024.2359641

Kovacevic, K., Tu, E., Rosen, N. O., Raposo, S., & Muise, A. (2024). Is spontaneous sex ideal? Beliefs and perceptions of spontaneous and planned sex and sexual satisfaction in romantic relationships. *Journal of Sex Research, 61*(2), 246–260. https://doi.org/10.1080/00224499.2022.2163611

Kowalczyk, R., Kaluga, M., Jacek, K., & Nowosielski, K. (2017). Sexual excitation, sexual inhibition, and prevalence of sexual disorders among MSM and heterosexual men. *European Psychiatry, 41*(S1), S850. https://doi.org/10.1016/j.eurpsy.2017.01.1686

Krafft-Ebing, R. (1892). *Psychopathia sexualis, with especial reference to contrary sexual instinct: A medico-legal study* (C. G. Chaddock, Trans., 7th ed.). F. A. Davis Co.

Kraus, S. W., Gola, M., Grubbs, J. B., Kowalewska, E., Hoff, R. A., Lew-Starowicz, M., Martino, S., Shirk, S. D., & Potenza, M. N. (2020). Validation of a Brief Pornography Screen across multiple samples. *Journal of Behavioral Addictions, 9*(2), 259–271. https://doi.org/10.1556/2006.2020.00038

Kraus, S. W., Krueger, R. B., Briken, P., First, M. B., Stein, D. J., Kaplan, M. S., Voon, V., Abdo, C. H. N., Grant, J. E., Atalla, E., & Reed, G. M. (2018). Compulsive sexual behaviour disorder in the ICD-11. *World Psychiatry, 17*(1), 109–110. https://doi.org/10.1002/wps.20499

Krause, C. E. (2023). Sexual disorders and paraphilic interests, male: Fetishism. In T. K. Shackelford (Ed.), *Encyclopedia of sexual psychology and behavior* (pp. 1–4). Springer International Publishing. https://doi.org/10.1007/978-3-031-08956-5_87-1

Laumann, E. O., Paik, A., & Rosen, R. C. (1999). Sexual dysfunction in the United States: Prevalence and predictors. *JAMA, 281*(6), 537–544. https://doi.org/10.1001/jama.281.6.537

Leath, S., Jerald, M. C., Perkins, T., & Jones, M. K. (2021). A qualitative exploration of Jezebel stereotype endorsement and sexual behaviors among Black college women. *The Journal of Black Psychology, 47*(4–5), 244–283. https://doi.org/10.1177/0095798421997215

Leeners, B., Tschudin, S., Wischmann, T., & Kalaitzopoulos, D. R. (2023). Sexual dysfunction and disorders as a consequence of infertility: A systematic review and meta-analysis. *Human Reproduction Update, 29*(1), 95–125. https://doi.org/10.1093/humupd/dmac030

Lehmiller, J. J. (2015). A comparison of sexual health history and practices among monogamous and consensually nonmonogamous sexual partners. *Journal of Sexual Medicine, 12*(10), 2022–2028. https://doi.org/10.1111/jsm.12987

Leonhardt, N. D., Busby, D. M., & Willoughby, B. J. (2020). Sex guilt or sanctification? The indirect role of religiosity on sexual satisfaction. *Psychology of Religion and Spirituality, 12*(2), 213–222. https://doi.org/10.1037/rel0000245

Levay, S., & Valente, S. M. (2006). *Human sexuality* (2nd ed.). Sinauer Press.

Lilley, C., Willmott, D., Mojtahedi, D., & Labhardt, D. (2023). Intimate partner rape: A review of six core myths surrounding women's conduct and the consequences of intimate partner rape. *Social Sciences, 12*(1), Article 34. https://doi.org/10.3390/socsci12010034

Maarefi, G., Ahmadi, M. S., Hatami, A., & Rashidi, N. (2020). A critique on the usage of Mosher's Sexual Guilt Scale in psychology and psychiatry researches in Islamic societies: Cultural differences in the meaning of sexual guilt. *International Journal of Multicultural and Multireligious Understanding, 7*(1), 47–55. https://ijmmu.com/index.php/ijmmu/article/view/1258

MacIntosh, H. B. (2019). *Developmental couple therapy for complex trauma: A manual for therapists*. Routledge. https://doi.org/10.4324/9781315210940

MacIntosh, H. B. (2024). Developmental couple therapy for complex trauma: Results of an implementation pilot study. *Journal of Marital and Family Therapy, 50*(3), 545–566. https://doi.org/10.1111/jmft.12711

Manley, M. H., Diamond, L. M., & van Anders, S. M. (2015). Polyamory, monoamory, and sexual fluidity: A longitudinal study of identity and sexual trajectories. *Psychology of Sexual Orientation and Gender Diversity, 2*(2), 168–180. https://doi.org/10.1037/sgd0000098

Marcinkowska, U. M., Shirazi, T., Mijas, M., & Roney, J. R. (2023). Hormonal underpinnings of the variation in sexual desire, arousal, and activity throughout the menstrual cycle: A multifaceted approach. *The Journal of Sex Research, 60*(9), 1297–1303. https://doi.org/10.1080/00224499.2022.2110558

Masters, W. H., & Johnson, V. E. (1966). *Human sexual response*. Little, Brown and Company.

Masters, W. H., & Johnson, V. E. (1970). *Human sexual inadequacy*. Little, Brown and Company.

McCabe, M. P., Sharlip, I. D., Lewis, R., Atalla, E., Balon, R., Fisher, A. D., Laumann, E., Lee, S. W., & Segraves, R. T. (2016). Incidence and prevalence of sexual dysfunction in women and men: A consensus statement from the Fourth International Consultation on Sexual Medicine 2015. *Journal of Sexual Medicine, 13*(2), 144–152. https://doi.org/10.1016/j.jsxm.2015.12.034

McNulty, J. K., Wenner, C. A., & Fisher, T. D. (2016). Longitudinal associations among relationship satisfaction, sexual satisfaction, and frequency of sex in early marriage. *Archives of Sexual Behavior, 45*(1), 85–97. https://doi.org/10.1007/s10508-014-0444-6

Meana, M. (2010). Elucidating women's (hetero) sexual desire: Definitional challenges and content expansion. *Journal of Sex Research, 47*(2–3), 104–122. https://doi.org/10.1080/00224490903402546

Meana, M., & Hall, K. (2024). Sexual dysfunctions. In F. T. L. Leong, J. L. Callahan, J. Zimmerman, M. J. Constantino, & C. F. Eubanks (Eds.), *APA handbook of psychotherapy: Vol. 1. Theory-driven practice and disorder-driven practice* (pp. 471–488). American Psychological Association. https://doi.org/10.1037/0000353-027

Meana, M., Hall, K. S., & Binik, Y. M. (2020). Conclusion: Where is sex therapy going? In Y. M. Binik & K. S. K. Hall (Eds.), *Principles and practice of sex therapy* (5th ed., pp. 505–522). The Guilford Press.

Meston, C. M., & Buss, D. M. (2007). Why humans have sex. *Archives of Sexual Behavior, 36*(4), 477–507. https://doi.org/10.1007/s10508-007-9175-2

Meston, C. M., Hamilton, L. D., & Harte, C. B. (2009). Sexual motivation in women as a function of age. *Journal of Sexual Medicine, 6*(12), 3305–3319. https://doi.org/10.1111/j.1743-6109.2009.01489.x

Meston, C. M., & Stanton, A. M. (2017). Recent findings on women's motives for engaging in sexual activity. *Current Sexual Health Reports, 9*(3), 128–135. https://doi.org/10.1007/s11930-017-0114-5

Miller, S. A., & Byers, E. S. (2012). Practicing psychologists' sexual intervention self-efficacy and willingness to treat sexual issues. *Archives of Sexual Behavior, 41*(4), 1041–1050. https://doi.org/10.1007/s10508-011-9877-3

Mintz, L. B. (2017). *Becoming cliterate: Why orgasm equality matters—And how to get it*. HarperOne.

Montejo, A. L., de Alarcón, R., Prieto, N., Acosta, J. M., Buch, B., & Montejo, L. (2021). Management strategies for antipsychotic-related sexual dysfunction: A clinical approach. *Journal of Clinical Medicine, 10*(2), 308–326. https://doi.org/10.3390/jcm10020308

Morin, J. (1995). *The erotic mind: Unlocking the inner sources of sexual passion and fulfillment*. HarperCollins.

Moser, C., & Kleinplatz, P. J. (2020). Conceptualization, history, and future of the paraphilias. *Annual Review of Clinical Psychology, 16*(1), 379–399. https://doi.org/10.1146/annurev-clinpsy-050718-095548

Mosher, D. L. (1966). The development and multitrait-multimethod matrix analysis of three measures of three aspects of guilt. *Journal of Consulting Psychology, 30*(1), 25–29. https://doi.org/10.1037/h0022905

Mosher, D. L. (2019). Revised Mosher Guilt Inventory. In R. R. Milhausen, J. K. Sakaluk, T. D. Fisher, C. M. Davis, & W. L. Yarber (Eds.), *Handbook of sexuality-related measures* (pp. 50–55). Routledge. https://doi.org/10.4324/9781315183169

Murray, S. H., Milhausen, R. R., Graham, C. A., & Kuczynski, L. (2017). A qualitative exploration of factors that affect sexual desire among men aged 30 to 65 in long-term relationships. *Journal of Sex Research*, *54*(3), 319–330. https://doi.org/10.1080/00224499.2016.1168352

Nagoski, E. (2021). *Come as you are: The surprising new science that will transform your sex life* (Rev. ed.). Simon & Schuster.

Nichols, M. (2013). Same-sex sexuality from a global perspective. In K. S. K. Hall & C. A. Graham (Eds.), *The cultural context of sexual pleasure and problems* (pp. 23–47). Routledge.

Nimbi, F. M., Appia, C., Tanzilli, A., Giovanardi, G., & Lingiardi, V. (2024). Deepening sexual desire and erotic fantasies research in the ACE spectrum: Comparing the experiences of asexual, demisexual, gray-asexual, and questioning people. *Archives of Sexual Behavior*, *53*(3), 1031–1045. https://doi.org/10.1007/s10508-023-02784-3

Nimbi, F. M., Ciocca, G., Limoncin, E., Fontanesi, L., Uysal, Ü. B., Flinchum, M., Tambelli, R., Jannini, E. A., & Simonelli, C. (2020). Sexual desire and fantasies in the LGBT+ community: Focus on lesbian women and gay men. *Current Sexual Health Reports*, *12*(3), 153–161. https://doi.org/10.1007/s11930-020-00263-7

Nobre, P. J., Carvalho, J., & Mark, K. P. (2020). Low sexual desire in men. In K. S. K. Hall & Y. M. Binik (Eds.), *Principles and practice of sex therapy* (6th ed., pp. 63–86). The Guilford Press.

Noll, J. G. (2021). Child sexual abuse as a unique risk factor for the development of psychopathology: The compounded convergence of mechanisms. *Annual Review of Clinical Psychology*, *17*(1), 439–464. https://doi.org/10.1146/annurev-clinpsy-081219-112621

North American Menopause Society. (n.d.-a). *Changes in the vagina and vulva*. The Menopause Society. Retrieved August 25, 2024, from https://www.menopause.org/for-women/sexual-health-menopause-online/changes-at-midlife/changes-in-the-vagina-and-vulva

North American Menopause Society. (n.d.-b). *Vaginal discomfort*. The Menopause Society. Retrieved February 10, 2025, from https://www.menopause.org/for-women/sexual-health-menopause-online/causes-of-sexual-problems/vaginal-discomfort

Ortmann, D. (2020). The pleasure of power. In K. S. K. Hall & Y. M. Binik (Eds.), *Principles and practice of sex therapy* (6th ed., pp. 294–316). The Guilford Press.

Oxford Languages. (n.d.). Surviving. In *Google dictionary*. Retrieved March 31, 2025, from https://www.google.com/search?client=firefox-b-1-d&q=surviving+definition

Pavanello Decaro, S., Portolani, D. M., Toffoli, G., Prunas, A., & Anzani, A. (2023). "There is no one way to be transgender and to live sex": Transgender and non-binary individuals' experiences with pornography. *Journal of Sex Research*, *61*(8), 1222–1232. https://doi.org/10.1080/00224499.2023.2215228

Perel, E. (2006). *Mating in captivity: Reconciling the erotic and the domestic*. Harper Collins.

Perel, E. (2017). *The state of affairs: Rethinking infidelity—A book for anyone who has ever loved*. Harper Collins.

Peterson, Z. D., & Buday, S. K. (2020). Sexual coercion in couples with infertility: Prevalence, gender differences, and associations with psychological outcomes. *Sexual and Relationship Therapy, 35*(1), 30–45. https://doi.org/10.1080/14681994.2018.1435863

Peterson, Z. D., Janssen, E., Goodrich, D., Fortenberry, J. D., Hensel, D. J., & Heiman, J. R. (2018). Child sexual abuse and negative affect as shared risk factors for sexual aggression and sexual HIV risk behavior in heterosexual men. *Archives of Sexual Behavior, 47*(2), 465–480. https://doi.org/10.1007/s10508-017-1079-1

Pulverman, C. S., Kilimnik, C. D., & Meston, C. M. (2018). The impact of childhood sexual abuse on women's sexual health: A comprehensive review. *Sexual Medicine Reviews, 6*(2), 188–200. https://doi.org/10.1016/j.sxmr.2017.12.002

Pulverman, C. S., & Meston, C. M. (2020). Sexual dysfunction in women with a history of childhood sexual abuse: The role of sexual shame. *Psychological Trauma: Theory, Research, Practice, and Policy, 12*(3), 291–299. https://doi.org/10.1037/tra0000506

Ross, M., Roijer, P., Mullender, M., & Grift, T. C. V. (2024). Trans, gender non-conforming and non-binary individuals' perspectives on experienced sexuality during medical transition. *Journal of Sex & Marital Therapy, 50*(3), 379–394. https://doi.org/10.1080/0092623X.2023.2300828

Rothmore, J. (2020). Antidepressant-induced sexual dysfunction. *The Medical Journal of Australia, 212*(7), 329–334. https://doi.org/10.5694/mja2.50522

Rubel, A. N., & Burleigh, T. J. (2020). Counting polyamorists who count: Prevalence and definitions of an under-researched form of consensual nonmonogamy. *Sexualities, 23*(1–2), 3–27. https://doi.org/10.1177/1363460718779781

Schild, S. M., Moore, A. S., Mattera, E. F., Fitzpatrick, M., Entezar, T., Fram, G., & Ching, T. H. (2024). Sexual orientation-themed obsessive-compulsive disorder in a lesbian woman: Phenomenology and implications for affirmative assessment and treatment. *Psychiatry Research Case Reports, 3*(1), 100211. Advance online publication. https://doi.org/10.1016/j.psycr.2024.100211

Seabra, D., Gato, J., Petrocchi, N., & do Céu Salvador, M. (2023). Shame experiences and psychopathology: The mediating role of self-compassion and social support in sexual minority individuals. *Journal of Evidence-Based Psychotherapies, 23*(1), 137–152. https://doi.org/10.24193/jebp.2023.1.6

Sexual desire: The real female orgasm. (2009, August 14). *Oprah.com*. Retrieved March 1, 2025, from https://www.oprah.com/relationships/sexual-desire-the-real-female-orgasm/all

Sheff, E. (2021, February 25). Polysaturation: When polyamorous people have enough partners. *Psychology Today*. https://www.psychologytoday.com/ca/blog/the-polyamorists-next-door/202102/polysaturation-when-polyamorous-people-have-enough-partners

Singer, B., & Toates, F. M. (1987). Sexual motivation. *Journal of Sex Research, 23*(4), 481–501. https://doi.org/10.1080/00224498709551386

Smith, A., Lyons, A., Ferris, J., Richters, J., Pitts, M., Shelley, J., & Simpson, J. M. (2011). Sexual and relationship satisfaction among heterosexual men and women: The importance of desired frequency of sex. *Journal of Sex & Marital Therapy, 37*(2), 104–115. https://doi.org/10.1080/0092623X.2011.560531

Steinberg, A., Alpert, J. L., & Courtois, C. A. (Eds.). (2021). Sexual boundary violations in the psychotherapy setting: An overview. In A. Steinberg, J. L. Alpert, & C. A. Courtois (Eds.), *Sexual boundary violations in psychotherapy: Facing therapist indiscretions, transgressions, and misconduct* (pp. 3–18). American Psychological Association. https://doi.org/10.1037/0000247-001

Stephenson, K. R., Ahrold, T. K., & Meston, C. M. (2011). The association between sexual motives and sexual satisfaction: Gender differences and categorical comparisons. *Archives of Sexual Behavior, 40*(3), 607–618. https://doi.org/10.1007/s10508-010-9674-4

Tiefer, L. (2004). *Sex is not a natural act & other essays*. Westview Press.

Underwood, R. (Director). (1991). *City Slickers* [Film]. Columbia Pictures.

Vaillancourt-Morel, M. P., Rosen, N. O., Štulhofer, A., Bosisio, M., & Bergeron, S. (2021). Pornography use and sexual health among same-sex and mixed-sex couples: An event-level dyadic analysis. *Archives of Sexual Behavior, 50*(2), 667–681. https://doi.org/10.1007/s10508-020-01839-z

van Anders, S. M. (2012). Testosterone and sexual desire in healthy women and men. *Archives of Sexual Behavior, 41*(6), 1471–1484. https://doi.org/10.1007/s10508-012-9946-2

Varod, S., Stern, A., Bőthe, B., & Gewirtz-Meydan, A. (2024). Who finds pornography stressful? A latent profile analysis. *Archives of Sexual Behavior, 53*(9), 3393–3404. Advance online publication. https://doi.org/10.1007/s10508-024-02927-0

Veale, D., Miles, S., Bramley, S., Muir, G., & Hodsoll, J. (2015). Am I normal? A systematic review and construction of nomograms for flaccid and erect penis length and circumference in up to 15,521 men. *BJU International, 115*(6), 978–986. https://doi.org/10.1111/bju.13010

Vedantu. (2024). Formula for the number of images formed by two plane mirrors. Retrieved August 25, 2024, from https://www.vedantu.com/jee-main/formula-for-number-of-images-formed-by-two-plane-physics-question-answer

Villeneuve, É., Paradis, A., Brassard, A., Vaillancourt-Morel, M. P., Fernet, M., Gewirtz-Meydan, A., & Godbout, N. (2024). Dissociation and sexual concerns in male survivors of childhood sexual abuse: The role of identity cohesion. *Journal of Trauma & Dissociation, 25*(4), 500–515. https://doi.org/10.1080/15299732.2024.2356597

Waldinger, M. D., Quinn, P., Dilleen, M., Mundayat, R., Schweitzer, D. H., & Boolell, M. (2005). A multinational population survey of intravaginal ejaculation latency time. *Journal of Sexual Medicine, 2*(4), 492–497. https://doi.org/10.1111/j.1743-6109.2005.00070.x

Wang, G. A., Corsini-Munt, S., Dubé, J. P., McClung, E., & Rosen, N. O. (2023). Regulate and communicate: Associations between emotion regulation and sexual communication among men with hypoactive sexual desire disorder and their partners. *Journal of Sex Research, 60*(3), 325–335. https://doi.org/10.1080/00224499.2022.2092588

Wang, Y., Fu, Y., Ghazi, P., Gao, Q., Tian, T., Kong, F., Zhan, S., Liu, C., Bloom, D. E., & Qiao, J. (2022). Prevalence of intimate partner violence against infertile women in low-income and middle-income countries: A systematic review and meta-analysis. *The Lancet Global Health, 10*(6), e820–e830. https://doi.org/10.1016/S2214-109X(22)00098-5

Warach, B., & Josephs, L. (2021). The aftershocks of infidelity: A review of infidelity-based attachment trauma. *Sexual and Relationship Therapy, 36*(1), 68–90. https://doi.org/10.1080/14681994.2019.1577961

Ward, T. (2002). Good lives and the rehabilitation of offenders: Promises and problems. *Aggression and Violent Behavior, 7*(5), 513–528. https://doi.org/10.1016/S1359-1789(01)00076-3

Watson, J. B. (1930). Review of *A research in marriage* by G. V. Hamilton and of *What is wrong with marriage?* by G. V. Hamilton & K. Macgowan. *The Journal of Social Psychology, 1*(1), 178–182.

Watter, D. (2023). *The existential importance of the penis*. Routledge. https://doi.org/10.4324/9781003127871

Watter, D. N. (2022). Keeping secrets in couples' sex therapy: Clinical and ethical considerations: Secrets in couples' sex therapy. *Journal of Sexual Medicine, 19*(12), 1721–1724. https://doi.org/10.1016/j.jsxm.2022.08.002

Wegmann, E., Antons, S., Schmidt, L. D., Klein, L., Montag, C., Rumpf, H. J., Müller, S. M., & Brand, M. (2025). Feels good, and less bad: Problematic use of the internet is associated with heightened experiences of both gratification and compensation. *Journal of Behavioral Addictions*, 1–13. https://doi.org/10.1556/2006.2024.00067

Weiner, L., & Avery-Clark, C. (2014). Sensate focus: Clarifying the Masters and Johnson's model. *Sexual and Relationship Therapy, 29*(3), 307–319. https://doi.org/10.1080/14681994.2014.892920

Weiner, L., & Avery-Clark, C. (2017). *Sensate focus in sex therapy: The illustrated manual*. Routledge. https://doi.org/10.4324/9781315630038

Weiser, D. A., Shrout, M. R., Thomas, A. V., Edwards, A. L., & Pickens, J. C. (2023). "I've been cheated, been mistreated, when will I be loved": Two decades of infidelity research through an intersectional lens. *Journal of Social and Personal Relationships, 40*(3), 856–898. https://doi.org/10.1177/02654075221113032

Weitzman, G. (2007). Counseling bisexuals in polyamorous relationships. In B. A. Firestein (Ed.), *Becoming visible: Counseling bisexuals across the lifespan* (pp. 312–335). Columbia University Press.

West, C. M. (1995). Mammy, Sapphire, and Jezebel: Historical images of black women and their implications for psychotherapy. *Psychotherapy: Theory,*

Research, & Practice, 32(3), 458–466. https://doi.org/10.1037/0033-3204.32.3.458

Williams, M. T., Wetterneck, C., Tellawi, G., & Duque, G. (2015). Domains of distress among people with sexual orientation obsessions. *Archives of Sexual Behavior, 44*(3), 783–789. https://doi.org/10.1007/s10508-014-0421-0

Williams, M. T., & Wetterneck, C. T. (2019). *Sexual obsessions in obsessive-compulsive disorder: A step-by-step, definitive guide to understanding, diagnosis, and treatment*. Oxford University Press. https://doi.org/10.1093/med-psych/9780190624798.001.0001

Wolpe, J. R. (1958). *Psychotherapy by reciprocal inhibition*. Stanford University Press.

Wolpe, J. R., & Lazarus, A. A. (1966). *Behavior therapy techniques*. Pergamon Press.

World Health Organization. (2019). *International statistical classification of diseases and related health problems* (11th ed.). https://icd.who.int/en

Yalom, I. D. (2002). *The gift of therapy: An open letter to a new generation of therapists and their patients*. Harper Perennial.

Zeglin, R. J., Goldberg, S., Stalnaker-Shofner, D. M., Walker, B. M., & Schubert, A. M. (2024). Sex therapy credentials: A descriptive analysis of the training of clinicians who do sex therapy. *Sexual and Relationship Therapy, 39*(1), 4–19. https://doi.org/10.1080/14681994.2021.1937598

Zeglin, R. J., Niemela, D. R. M., & Vandenberg, M. (2019). What does the counseling field say about sexuality? A content analysis. *American Journal of Sexuality Education, 14*(1), 55–73. https://doi.org/10.1080/15546128.2018.1518175

Index

A

K

L

M

R

S

T

U

V

W

Y

Z

About the Author

Kathryn S. K. Hall, PhD, received her doctorate from McGill University in Montreal, Canada. A licensed psychologist with over 4 decades of experience in sex therapy, she has coedited three influential books: two editions of *Principles and Practice of Sex Therapy* and *The Cultural Context of Sexual Pleasure and Problems: Psychotherapy With Diverse Clients*. Dr. Hall has authored a popular book on female sexual desire, *Reclaiming Your Sexual Self: How You Can Bring Desire Back Into Your Life*, which won the SSTAR Consumer Book Award in 2006. Dr. Hall takes great pride in providing sex therapy training to aspiring and seasoned clinicians alike. She is the book review editor for the *Journal of Sex and Marital Therapy* and is a past president of the Society for Sex Therapy and Research. Visit https://drkathrynhall.com/ to learn more about Dr. Hall.